THE SCIENCE OF
HIGHER SENSE PERCEPTION

The Science of
Higher Sense Perception

R. EUGENE NICHOLS

Parker Publishing Company, Inc.   West Nyack, N.Y.

Library of Congress Cataloging in Publication Data

Nichols, R   Eugene.
  The science of higher sense perception.

  1. Senses and sensation. 2. Psychology, Applied.
I. Title.
BF233.N5   131.3   72-5405
ISBN 0-13-795443-3

Dedicated to my daughters, Lynette and Celeste

What This Book
Can Do For You

In this book you will step with me into a new dimension of sense perception—a dimension of expanded mental and psychic powers. Within you, as well as every person, are powers you have never tapped. A systematic understanding of these powers can lift you to new levels of happiness, security, and material abundance, give you greater freedom, guide you, protect you, and set your feet upon the highway to successful and masterful living.

How do you tap these powers? By discovering the *higher* reaches of the senses you now possess . . . by developing your latent *higher sense perception* or HSP. In the pages that follow, I shall share with you simplified, systematic techniques which enable adults and teenagers alike to turn psychic potentials into practical powers for successful living.

WHAT HIGHER SENSORY POWERS
HAVE DONE FOR OTHERS

Through a quarter of a century I have lectured and written on higher sensory powers, and I have witnessed transformations in the lives of countless people who have recognized and used these expanded powers of mind consciously. The changes they demonstrated, you can also experience, for example:

—Totally new ability to solve daily problems to your satisfaction
—Protection and an amazing sense of security in daily affairs
—Success and abundance of material riches

—Friends and desirable companionship

—Health of mind and body

—Freedom from the specters of fear that are choking your success

—New self-command over your destiny and ability to influence others

—Peace of mind in a changing world to meet all challenges thrown at you

The age when psychic powers were mere curiosities and stage-show gimmicks is gone. There is a growing awareness today that telepathy, clairvoyance, clairaudience, precognition, and teleki-nesis are genuine powers which every individual possesses in some degree. Extra-sensory perception for example is not to be ridiculed or spoken of in whispers behind drawn curtains. It is to be practiced openly and confidently on the great stage of daily life, HSP is to be used for your successful, expanded living to secure all that you ever wanted for yourself.

HOW YOU CAN USE THIS BOOK

How can you make the most of this book? Read it with the attitude that you wish to find something totally new and exciting for masterful living. Use it as a tool to develop the higher sensory powers potential within you. It contains twenty PSI-PRO-GRAMMING POINTERS to help you program your mind with an expanded self-image. The PSI term in PSI-PROGRAMMING POINTERS indicates the dynamic factors of psychic or parapsy-chological powers available to energize your programs and bring them to a successful conclusion. There are also 10 HSP SENSI-TIVITY TRAINING TECHNIQUES.

These TRAINING TECHNIQUES awaken in you sleeping powers that can remake your life the way you want to live it. They lead you in the development of telepathy. They guide you in the use of directed-dream power. They help you break the time-barrier that may stand between you and success. They help you tap precognitive and retrocognitive powers, enabling you to perceive future business trends and past motives. They attune you to the cosmic radiant of health. Finally, the TRAINING TECH-NIQUES lead you in an understanding of life beyond this time and place through laws of recurrence and rebirth.

Throughout the pages of this book run the higher mental

laws—Laws of the Science of Higher Sense Perception—you can use to demonstrate a successful life and dispel any sense of bewilderment, self-dissatisfaction, feeling of inadequacy. or frustration you may have.

I do not present this volume with the claim that it is the final word on a subject which is as big as life itself, I do assert, however, that the simplified science its pages reveal will expand your mind, deepen your awareness, and equip you as you may never have been previously to have and to hold anything and everything you want with your new-found use of HSP powers.

R. Eugene Nichols

Your Guide to Psi-Power

Here is the way to unfold the powers hidden within your mind! After you have read this book once, continue to expand your psi-ability by turning to the page listed for a specific Psi-Programming Pointer. Read the paragraphs that introduce it. This refreshes for you the purpose of the pointer. Then, copy it and let its significance sink into your subconscious mind, becoming a part of your self-image.

1. To activate the superior wisdom latent within you, use: Psi-Programming Pointer on page 18.

2. To put yourself in a favored position where extended sensory powers are normal, use: Psi-Programming Pointer on page 26.

3. To reach that radiant level of consciousness where health and happiness abound, use: Psi-Programming Pointer on page 38.

4. To think on-key and put yourself in tune with the cosmic radiant, apply: Psi-Programming Pointer on page 48.

5. To screen out psychic messages that are false and become a meta-seer, use: Psi-Programming Pointer on page 60.

6. To prepare yourself psychologically for success in demonstrating higher sensory powers, use: Psi-Programming Pointer on page 70.

7. To get the "BIG VIEW" that defies past, present, and future, apply: Psi-Programming Pointer on page 81.

8. To gain retrocognitive insight into past motives and the cause of things, use: Psi-Programming Pointer on page 86.

9   To develop a listening attitude and attune yourself to telepathic psi-phone reception, use: Psi-Programming Pointer on page 102.

10. To connect with the success circuits of others on the universal mental switchboard, use: Psi-Programming Pointer on page 106.

11. To explore the reaches of the subconscious mind through automatic writing, use: Psi-Programming Pointer on page 119.

12. To keep your psychic development directed toward constructive and safe results, practice: Psi-Programming Pointer on page 126.

13. To become master of your emotions and guide them wisely in the waking state and dream state, use: Psi-Programming Pointer on page 143.

14. To retain the power of choice and avoid unwanted psychic experiences, practice: Psi-Programming Pointer on page 163.

15. To invoke vibrations of love and harmony in your environment, apply: Psi-Programming Pointer on page 167.

16. To overcome a dull, negative aura that turns friends and success away, use: Psi-Programming Pointer on page 181.

17. To protect yourself from "sappers" and generate a vigorous success aura, use: Psi-Programming Pointer on page 184.

18. To build a positive aura-lux that repels undesirable influences, practice: Psi-Programming Pointer on page 186.

19. To change your response-pattern and break the hold of negative memories, use: Psi-Programming Pointer on page 202.

20. To experience an incarnation of freedom and expanded sensory powers, practice: Psi-Programming Pointer on page 205.

CONTENTS

1

How Your Discovery of HSP
(Higher Sense Perception)
Can Change Your Life

"You must be psychic!"
"I had a feeling I shouldn't have gone!"
"You took the words right out of my mouth!"
"I can read her like an open book."
"I just knew it would happen!"
"I've been thinking about you all day."
"You must have been reading my mind!"
"How did you know what I was thinking?"
"I had the strangest feeling about that!"

These are but a few of the statements I have heard people make who never dreamed they had psychic powers.

People have hunches, they get telepathic messages, they know things intuitively, a parade of psychic experiences march through their lives, but they seldom recognize them as extra-sensory events.

How psychic are you?

How psychic are you? Don't say you aren't, for everyone has powers over and above the normal level of sense perception.

Everyone has an extension of the objective powers of seeing, smelling, feeling, tasting, and hearing

You will discover as you read on that you have already had experiences that can be classified as instances of higher sense perception (HSP). You will also discover as you use the techniques in this book that you can tune into feelings of others, converse with friends by non-physical means, tap wisdom-wells of knowledge, probe past motives, perceive future trends in business, dial success circuits when dealing with other people, use directed-dream power for decisions, stop the cyclicon of recurring failure, and explore the mystic level of the superconscious.

Do you think this is impossible? Impossible things are happening every day. Men are flying to the moon, probing other planets, photographing past events, broadcasting by telestar, and the list goes on and on. No one now says, "such things are impossible." This is because they have already been demonstrated. Once you demonstrate the expanded powers taught in this book, you'll no longer say of psychic experience, "That is impossible."

Are you a believer or a skeptic? If you are a skeptic, good! Don't put this book aside. Because believer and skeptic alike can benefit from the disclosures in these pages on ways to develop, expand, cultivate, and extend the higher sense powers that are latent within everyone.

This book is a tool!

This book is to be used, not merely read. It is a tool. Use it to discover the higher powers of your mind and to put those powers to work! Between these covers are training techniques that will change your life for the better. Utilize them to demonstrate knowledge, insight, vision, judgment, protection, financial freedom, personal attainment, and success by expansion of the psychic aspect of your mind.

Don't be one to say, "Oh, *I'm* not psychic, but I've known of people who are." I have news for you. You *are* psychic. And, through your use and faithful practice of the PSI-PROGRAMMING POINTERS and HSP SENSITIVITY TRAINING TECHNIQUES incoporated in the following pages, you will come out on the other side of this book a bigger person than you ever dreamed of being.

Your mind will be stretched and expanded to include higher dimensions of experience, and a mind so stretched can never return to its previous size. You will be not just a renewed person—you will be a *new person!*

What is a Psi-Programming Pointer?

First, consider the meaning of the term *psi.* By dictionary definition, it is the twenty-third letter of the Greek alphabet—the symbol **Ψ**. This symbol will be used to designate the Psi-Programming Pointers in this book.

Psi, as used in the Science of Higher Sense Perception and in parapsychology, represents the *invisible* or behind-the-scenes forces that underlie the *visible* aspects of life. The term *psi* includes reference to various psychic phenomena such as telepathy, clairvoyance, clairaudience, precognition, retrocognition, psycho-kinesis, intuition, etc.

Psi, therefore, may be defined as an abbreviation for the term *psychic power.* It is an ability possessed by all life. The *homing sense* of a pigeon, the *radar perception* of a bat, the mysteries of *pathfinding* in wild creatures, and *higher sense perception* at all levels of life may rightly be termed *psi-ability.*

A Psi-Programming Pointer is a statement of truth about your psi-ability. It is a declaration about the *potentialities* in you that you wish to make into *actualities.* When such a statement is programmed into the deeper level of the subconscious mind, it becomes a dynamo of creative power for you. It changes your self-image. It turns your potentialities into actualities!

A Psi-Programming Pointer is more than a few words to repeat by rote. The meaning of the words must trigger a belief in the depths of your being. The pointers must trigger a feeling-response. As you repeat them, they must make you *feel* a sense of excitement and expectancy. For this reason, they cannot be spoken once and idly forgotten. They must be used repeatedly. Regular use is the process of *programming.* The more the statement on the Psi-Pointer is repeated, the greater is its impression on the subconscious mind.

A computer program consists of a series of statements setting forth the operations that the computer is to perform. Likewise, Psi-Programming Pointers are a series of statements setting forth the operations you wish the subconscious mind to perform. To register effectively in the subsconscious, the pointers must be read and re-read. Put the one you are working on some place where you will see it several times a day—on the bedroom mirror, near the kitchen sink, on the dashboard of your car, or some other obvious place.

The "programming" comes from reading the statement often so that the inner level of the subconscious mind is impressed and activated. That inner mind is creative and will manifest the images you give it, once they are fed into it.

How to test your Psi-ability

One of the first Psi-Programming Pointers I give to members joining an HSP class is on protection and guidance. Not only does it serve to guide a person around physical mishaps, it helps him understand the new techniques he is encountering.

Here it is . . . your first Psi-Programming Pointer designed to help guide you in applying the HSP techniques disclosed in this book. It is a statement about yourself. You may feel on first reading that it is not a true statement about you. But remember, it is like a set of computer directions. *Program it into the subconscious, and let the subconscious make it true!*

The statement deals with your intellect and with the fact that there is *something superior* to it. There must be something that makes your intellect possible. How can there be intellect unless there is a source of that intellect—a reservoir from which it springs! It is this larger reservoir of knowledge and guidance, this superior source, you tap as you work with the following Psi-Programming Pointer.

Test your psi-ability now. Repeat the statement three times. Then, make a copy of it and keep it with you. Program it into the deep, creative center of your consciousness, and you will be surprised to find yourself *learning* and *mastering* the techniques of Higher Sense Perception.

Ψ   Psi-Programming Pointer
THERE IS A WISDOM SUPERIOR TO MY CONSCIOUS INTELLECT THAT GUIDES MY EVERY ACTION. I LISTEN AND I LEARN. I KEEP EVER ALERT TO THIS NEW SOURCE OF KNOWLEDGE AND GUIDANCE.

Steve was a skeptic until .

"I just can't buy that," Steve declared. He was one of several members who had just joined my class in HSP development. We were chatting informally after the first lesson, and someone mentioned an out-of-the-body experience. Steve turned away in disbelief.

Later Steve cornered me, "Do you think I should continue with this class?" he asked. "I listen to you but so many unanswered questions crowd in."

"Questions are fine! It shows you're thinking. You're the kind of person I welcome in an HSP class, Steve, and I promise your questions will be answered as this Science unfolds."

Steve was skeptical! He was not, however, antagonistic. He just wanted to be convinced with logical, acceptable reasoning. According to him, he'd never had a psychic experience. But, he was open-minded, and this is the only real requirement for the person who wants to learn HSP techniques.

As the weeks passed, Steve continued to ask "why" and "how" about the working of psi-powers. His remarks remained somewhat critical when others talked about experiences that seemed *far out,* especially when they were based only on hearsay. Steve wanted things explained logically in terms of how and why.

It is this urge to know *how* and *why* that has sparked the most exciting thinking mankind has done. Of course, it is much easier to explain the *how* of things, than the *why*. In natural science, most of the research carried on is devoted to how things happen. For example, in dealing with the laws of polarity and motion, the scientist can easily explain *how* two bodies attract each other, but it is harder to explain *why*.

Why is this? It is because man is finite and the universe is infinite. The finite will never be able to completely explain the Infinite. *The finite is confined to an explanation of the finite workings of the Infinite!* Man, by observing, can grasp *the how* of that working, and, by inference, he can deduce *the why*.

This is what is done in the Science of Higher Sense Perception. The many techniques, devices, and training exercises given demonstrate *how* higher sense powers work, and the theories infer the reason *why* they work. The techniques are systematic. They unfold scientifically. They take the guesswork out of the discovery and use of psi-power for fulfillment, happiness and success.

Steve was quite willing to develop whatever HSP powers he could, in spite of his persistent "hows" and "whys". He did practice the Psi-Programming Pointers and HSP Sensitivity Training Techniques. However, his skeptical attitude finally piqued another class member who demanded, "Steve, why do you try to practice it if you don't believe in it?"

"When you are in a class, you should do what you are supposed to do or you shouldn't be there," was his simple reply.

Steve's faithful application paid off shortly and turned him from a skeptic into a believer.

An experience in psychic protection

Toward the middle of the class series, Steve missed a night, and I felt something had happened. When he returned, he surprised us all during the workshop period. For once, instead of asking questions, he had an account to tell! It was his first psychic experience!

Steve told of a dream that he'd had for three successive nights. Each repeat was substantially the same. "In the dream," Steve related, "I was driving down a dark canyon road. It was the same road each time, with variations. In one dream, a bridge was washed out on the road; in the second, the road came to an abrupt dead-end; in the third, there was a rock-slide blocking the road."

At the end of each dream, Steve explained, he awoke startled with these words ringing in his ears: "I told you not to come."

"These dreams occurred," Steve continued, "about the time I was invited to attend a football game in a nearby college town with some friends. I had the dreams on Sunday, Monday, and Tuesday. The game wasn't until Saturday. As the day grew nearer, the feeling that I shouldn't go grew stronger On Saturday, I called my friend and told him I wasn't going. I hardly knew why I did it, but I didn't have to wait long to find out."

Steve swallowed hard, "My friends met with an accident on the way to the game. As their car rounded a bend, it hit a large boulder that had fallen from the canyon wall. Their car was thrown off the road, and it rolled down an embankment killing the boy I had called. The two others in the car were badly injured."

"I am convinced," Steve said, "that my dreams were a form of psychic guidance and that the work I am doing with HSP protected me. I guess I was a skeptic before, but this really excites me."

Steve paused. "My deep regret is that I couldn't see far enough to help my friends. Why didn't I perceive that the trip would be a tragedy for them too?"

I explained to Steve that he had just begun to tap the psi-abilities potential to him and, although he had been working with the first Psi-Programming Pointer (the one you are already using for personal guidance), many other techniques yet lay ahead of him. One of those is the development of clairvoyance and the ability to demonstrate guidance for friends with whom you are en rapport (a technique you will find in Chapter Three).

Steve needed a greater grasp of his inner self before he delved further into psi-powers. He needed to know what made him tick, a knowledge essential to everyone who wishes to master the Science of Higher Sense Perception.

It's time to find out what makes you tick

Man, generally, is in the dark about his mind. He is a mystery unto himself. He doesn't know what makes him tick, but, if he is curious enough, he can find out.

I remember the curiosity that filled me when I received my first watch. It was a Christmas gift from my mother when I was a young boy. I was very proud of that watch. I was intrigued by its ticking, by the movement of the hands, and by the fact that it could keep time. What made the watch tick and how it was able to tell time was a mystery to me.

I could hardly wait to get the back off and observe more closely the activity that was going on. Of course, even with the back off I could only see the springs and the movement of the assorted wheels. But it gave me a feeling that I knew what was going on. This is what *you* need to do. You need to look inside yourself and become aware of the intricate mechanism of mind that makes you tick.

Compare the outside case of a watch to your physical self. The case is just the outer shell that houses the inner works. It is the visible House-of-Self in which an invisible YOU dwells. The outside of the case (the body) seems fairly simple. It has five sensory perceptors for seeing, smelling, tasting, feeling, and hearing. It has two arms, two legs, and the other standard equipment. But this equipment functions only because of what is inside—just like a watch.

Inside the case, the mysterious wheels of your mind click and turn, producing results that are a wonder to behold. Although the case (the body) has sense perceptors, the one who actually perceives is the tenant inside the House-of-Self. The real You is the one who sees, smells, tastes, feels, and hears.

You do not hear with your auditory nerve, you hear with your mind. You do not feel with tactile nerve endings, but with your mind. You do not see with your optic nerve, but with your mind. So it is with all the physical senses; *all* are actually mental processes.

Can it not be surmised that mental processes beyond those now used are potential to man? Can he become sensitive to stimuli he knows little about as yet? Can he improve his sensitivity to already-existing stimuli and expand his mental processes beyond the limited range of his present five senses? The Science of Higher Sense Perception says YES.

The HSP Sensitivity Training Techniques found in this book are designed to help you demonstrate a sensitivity to stimuli beyond the usual range of sight and sound. As you hear not with your ears but with your mind, you will find that it is possible to experience a hearing that is independent of the ear. As you see not with the eye but with the mind, you will find that it is possible to experience a vision that is independent of the eye.

As you develop a sensitivity that extends beyond the five senses, you will discover vast new dimensions about the real YOU—that inner tenant in the House-of-Self.

Your potentialities include ALL THINGS

The ancient Psalmist asked, "What is man that thou art mindful of him, and the son of man that thou visiteth him? For thou hast made him a little lower than the angels, and hast crowned him with glory and honour. Thou hast made him to have dominion over the works of thy hands; thou hast put *all things* under his feet."

What is included in *all things?* Is there anything that can really be excluded? What are the potentialities available to man? Up to now, man's powers have not embraced *all things*, so it is obvious that he has accepted self-limitations that do not rightfully belong to him.

All things, all powers, all mental potentialities belong *normally* to man. Some of these powers are commonplace. Other powers are less common for they are *above* average sense perception. When your mind uses these powers above average sense perception, mental scientists say that it is acting as a *Tele-Data Receiver*. That means that it is receiving psychic information through *above-average* sense receptors – not your sight or hearing, but much more powerful senses deep in the mind.

It is this above-average range of mental abilities that is dealt with in this book and termed *higher sensory perception.* Because this higher range of power is not abnormal to man, it is not *extra-*sensory. Each person is capable of tapping and utilizing it for more successful, dynamic living!

What do you believe to be normal?

What do you believe to be normal for you and your fellow man? Do you think that only powers presently in evidence are normal? Let's list the mental powers that today seem so typical and natural for man: he displays the power of reason, analysis, synthesis, discrimination, deduction, observation, perception, etc.

Were these mental powers *always* accepted as normal? Was the Neanderthal man capable of the advanced logic widely displayed today? Obviously, he was not. Yet, the potentiality for the development of advanced mental powers was within him.

What about a hundred years hence or a thousand? Will abilities not presently in evidence become standard equipment? Will they be accepted as normal? The answer given by the Science of Higher Sense Perception is a definite YES!

Just as powers of advanced logic were potential to the Neanderthal man, powers of higher sense perception are potential to man now. Advanced psi-powers are not abnormal or even extra-normal—*they are superbly normal.* The man who can expand his concept of normalcy and accept a superior self-image will find it normal to use superbly normal powers!

Until man does stretch upward in consciousness, however, his present *belief* in what is normal for him will tend to bind him to a familiar pattern of experience. Thomas Troward, the father of Mental Science, says: "We shall bring into manifestation the conditions corresponding to the sort of personality we accept as our normal standard . . . What we shall eventually attain is, not what we merely wish, but what we regard as normal."[1]

What you believe to be your *normal* range of sense perception will remain your range until you expand your beliefs. You may need to re-examine what you now regard to be within the mental scope of human experience. Perhaps you have given little thought to abilities that lie beyond the confines of the five familiar senses accepted as normal. If so, accept the possibility NOW that there are expanded senses beyond these five that are *just as natural* to man when he reaches a higher normalcy of expression.

Exploring a higher standard of normalcy

Was it normal for Joan of Arc to hear voices? Was it normal for Socrates to have his guiding "Daemon"? Was it normal for Calpurnia to have a disturbing dream prior to the death of her husband, Julius Caesar? Was it normal for Lincoln to have a dream of his own death six weeks before his assassination? Was it normal for Mark Twain (in a dream or vision) to see his brother lying in a coffin a short time before he was killed in a steamboat accident on the Mississippi?

Traditionally, these events, and the numerous experiences shared with you in the pages that follow, are regarded as

---

[1]Troward, Thomas, *The Creative Process in the Individual.* New York: Dodd, Mead & Company, 1949, p. 63.

abnormal. This is only because the *normal* standard is based upon a narrow understanding of man's total potentialities. The aim of this book is to build the framework for a higher standard of normalcy. Using this framework, you will be able to fashion an expanded standard for yourself which will enable you to accept as normal and natural such extended powers as telepathy, precognition, retrocognition, clairvoyance, clairaudience, and intuition.

Programming your mind for superbly normal powers

When the proposition came up one evening that superbly normal powers are potential to every man, Larry R., another class member, objected.

"It seems to me," he asserted, "that HSP powers are *extra-normal*—that they are the *exception* rather than the rule. Granted, there have been men and women through the ages who have demonstrated these powers, but they were unusual. How can you assume that psi-powers belong to everyone?"

Larry continued, "Every generation has had its tall minds who were favored with extra powers, but it also had a lot of clods. Are you suggesting that these clods can blossom forth with psi-abilities?"

I assured Larry and the class that every person can expand the powers of perception. "Take your remark," I said, "that certain ones have been especially favored. By whom, or by what, are they favored? Isn't it more accurate to assume that, rather than *being favored,* their expanded powers of mind sprang from the attitudes, self-images, and beliefs which *they favored?* They favored higher standards of normalcy, and their attitude sparked a corresponding experience!"

"Take this assumption," I suggested, "as a working hypothesis and prove it in your own experience."

At this point I gave Larry and the class a Psi-Programming Pointer similar to the following one which they were to use for the duration of their ten-week series. This they agreed to do. They *favored* the attitude that expanded powers were normal to them by programming that attitude into subconscious mind. This is the next step for you, too. Program the following statement of truth into your subconscious, letting the subconscious make it true in your experience.

Ψ   Psi-Programming Pointer
    EXTENDED SENSORY POWERS ARE AS NATURAL AND
    NORMAL AS MY FIVE SENSES. I NOW CLAIM THESE
    SUPERBLY NORMAL POWERS FOR MYSELF AND LET
    THEM MANIFEST AS EXPANDED ABILITY IN MY DAILY
    ENDEAVORS.

Examples of higher sense perception

The Science of Higher Sense Perception not only reveals the higher standard of normalcy you can attain, but it gives you techniques for developing the powers that belong to this higher standard. In the chapters to follow, you will see how these techniques accord with universal, scientific principles that support the reasonableness of higher sensory equipment.

For example, at the objective level, sound natural principles have been utilized in the invention of the telephone, telegraph, and short wave. All of these are devices that enable you to communicate with loved ones and friends at great distances.

If man is able to invent an objective telephone, then a universal principle of communication must already exist. The outward mechanical device mirrors an inward principle that is not exhausted or confined by man's present technology. Stated simply, the communication principal that man uses at the physical level as the telephone may be used at a higher level as telepathy.

If man is able to invent television, radar, sonar, X-ray, and the like, then universal principles underlying these inventions must exist. Man has been marvelous at conceiving and inventing mechanical representations of inner principles. What he needs to do now is to utilize on the non-objective level the same principles he has used to make so many ingenious objects on the physical level.

Without a doubt, you have already had some encounters with universal principles on the non-objective level. Perhaps you did not recognize them as HSP experiences. Perhaps you did, but kept them to yourself for fear that others would think you strange. It may have been a voice you heard that you could not explain, or a form you saw, or an unusual feeling you had prior to receiving critical news. Or, it may have been as simple a thing as thinking of someone and having the phone ring, only to find that it was the person of whom you were thinking.

For example, just the other day I saw a note on my desk calendar reminding me of a person I needed to call. I did not dial immediately, for other matters came along to interrupt. However, my mind kept going back to the note, and the thought recurred to me several times.

Finally, I reached for the phone to call, and, without the bell having rung even once, the voice of the person I was going to dial spoke to me. Within that split second after my friend had dialed, I too had picked up the telephone receiver to call. Such an occurrence is usually passed off as being a *coincidence*. But, does that explain anything?

This book is designed to give you undergirding principles that will help explain such *coincidences*. It will provide logical laws of mind that show how higher-sensory events take place. But more than that, it is the purpose of this Science to explain man from the standpoint of a higher normalcy to which extended powers are natural. With that knowledge, you will be able to develop your higher-sense-perception self and the extended powers you should normally enjoy . . . from that *higher* normalcy.

Learn to know yourself as part of Something bigger!

Although the finite cannot explain the Infinite in other than finite terms, the finite must try. Man must try to grasp the magnitude of the principles that undergird his being. For too long he has timidly embraced the *infinitesimal*, whereas he should be encompassing the *Infinite*.

Man must come to know himself as part of *Something bigger*. Just as a mathematical equation is part of something bigger—the principle of mathematics—so you are part of the principle of mind. Just as a chemical formula is part of something bigger—the principles of chemistry—so you are part of something bigger. This *Something* is the infinite source from which knowingness springs.

What is that infinite *Something* like? Man, being finite, can only define it by inference.

For example, take the principle of mathematics again. The combined laws of all known systems of mathematics—algebra, geometry, trigonometry, calculus, etc.—do not fully represent the limitless potentials of the principle itself. They represent only what man has discovered about how it works. Undreamed of theories of mathematics still lie untouched in the principle.

The same inference can be made about the principle of mind. The combined discoveries of all known systems of inquiry into the nature of man—genetics, anthropology, psychology, psychosomatics, mental cybernetics, philosophy, religion, etc.—do not fully represent the magnitude of the principle itself. They represent only what has been explained about man up to now.

Thus, it can be inferred that man has only scratched the surface of knowledge about himself and about his infinite source. To say that there are no potentials of power beyond man's present mental status is very much like a tadpole saying that the frog does not exist. Man's potentialities are *bigger* than he realizes.

The Sea of Universal Mind gave birth to you

The Science of Higher Sense Perception is premised upon the understanding that *something does not come out of nothing.* The mind of man must come out of a universal Mind that ever unfolds through individualized expression. This Science is also premised on the fact that *the part cannot be greater than the whole.* This Something—this source—from which the mind of man springs must be infinitely greater than man and must have always existed.

Dr. Alan W. Watts, in *The Book—On the Taboo Against Knowing Who You Are,* says, "We do not 'come into' this world; we come out of it, as leaves from a tree. As the ocean 'waves,' the universe 'peoples.' Every individual is an expression of the whole realm of nature, a unique action of the total universe."[2]

Mankind springs from an ocean of universal Mind, and all of the powers and potentialities belonging to that Mind are resident within each man. Just as a drop of sea water, if taken from the ocean and chemically analyzed, would contain the same properties as the ocean—the same salts, nitrates, minerals, etc.—the mind of man contains the same properties as universal Mind. Man has *come out of* universal Mind.

---

[2]Watts, Alan W., *The Book—On the Taboo Against Knowing Who You Are.* New York: Pantheon Books, a division of Random House, Inc., 1967, p. 6.

However, man is not *individual* (not separate) but *individualized*. He is an individualized expression. As a wave of the ocean can never be a wave by itself but is the *ocean as a wave,* so it is with man. Man is *universal-Mind-as-man.*

Of course, the individual may be a great tidal wave or a small ripple upon the surface of the Infinite. It is what man *does* with his individuality that makes him great or small and creates for him a heaven or a hell. Because man enjoys the same properties as the mental sea from which he comes, his thought is creative and his dreams mold his experience. As the poet writes, you live in a mental sea:

> Midst stone and flesh, you occupy
> A universe of thought—
> A mental sea of boundless range,
> A sphere both intimate and strange,
> Where swirling nuclei of mind
> Give form unto each dream designed.
> Where thought and cosmic substance merge,
> Initiate creation's surge,
> And toss upon the waiting sand
> The pearls or rubble you demand.
> There, *there* is where your life is swayed;
> There your heaven or hell is made!
> Yes, from a universe of thought
> The stone and flesh of earth are wrought. [3]

Universal Mind transcends man, as the ocean *transcends* the wave, but it is also imminent in man, as the ocean is *in* the wave. As man realizes this relationship, he grasps the significance of his potentialities. He is not separate from infinite Mind; he is an *individualization* of it. He is *one* with it.

This sense of *oneness* wipes out the feeling that to attain success he must incorporate something he does not now possess. This sense of *oneness* makes him aware that all he must do to succeed is to open the door to the gift that is already given. It is this sense of oneness that HSP Sensitivity Training Technique No. 1 is designed to awaken in you.

---

[3] Nichols, Winnifred, "Creation's Surge." From an unpublished collection of poems.

What is an HSP Sensitivity Training Technique?

The Sensitivity Training Techniques found at the close of each chapter differ somewhat from Psi-Programming Pointers. Each programmer pinpoints a specific HSP truth which is to be fed into the subconscious mind *for subsequent manifestation.* Sensitivity Training, on the other hand, is designed to produce an experience in consciousness *at the time it is practiced.*

Psi-Programming Pointers may be repeated during the day at brief times when the mind is idle. Sensitivity Training, on the other hand, cannot be approached as casually. It is more formal training, and you must take care to create a contemplative mood for it. It is designed to awaken your sensitivity to higher experiences in consciousness. As you use it, you will become aware of new sensations. New mental vistas will open up before you. You will become sensitive to higher-sensory stimuli.

Each HSP Sensitivity Training Technique is an exercise in mind-stretching. Before you begin it, read the technique over until you have almost memorized it. Then, put yourself through the training with your eyes closed, following its unfoldment step-by-step.

The initial one at the end of this chapter is designed to be a trip in mind-expansion, and its purpose is to make you keenly aware of your oneness with universal Mind—the source of power you will be tapping in this study.

This experience in consciousness-expansion awaiting you in each Sensitivity Training session is not to be confused with the experiments in mind-expansion induced by drugs. Drugs lead one into forced, *artificial* sensory experiences. In addition, lysergic acid diethylamid (LSD), hashish, marijuana, and other chemicals produce unpredictable effects upon the mental and emotional centers. Such trips may be good or bad. Very little, if anything, can be done to insure whether the experience will be terrifying or uplifting (a subject dealt with in more detail later.)

There is a way, however, to take a safe "trip" and that is through *natural* mind-expansion. Such is the trip you may take now to increase your sensitivity to *oneness* with universal Mind. This trip will be a good one, I can assure you. It will not wrest from your hands emotional control, nor will it have unpleasant side effects. True, the good you experience will be largely up to you. Your willingness, your attention to instructions, and your eager participation will bring rewards of inestimable value. You have nothing to lose and everything to gain.

HOW TO PREPARE FOR THE TRIP

First, select a room of your home where you will not be disturbed by others or interrupted by the ringing of the phone.

Second, choose a chair that is comfortable, but not so soft that you will fall asleep. It should be a chair that you can call your own, rather than one that is used by various members of your family. There is a reason for this which will be explained later.

Third, schedule an early morning hour for your psi-sensitivity training, if at all possible. It is important that your journey be close to the same time each day. If you cannot arrange your time thus, do not fight conditions. But conform, as closely as you can, to these rules.

Fourth, thoughtfully read and follow the instructions given next for opening the door of the mind to your oneness with life, as a realization of *oneness* is the necessary first step in developing your higher sensory powers. Then, close your eyes and put yourself through this sensitivity training step-by-step.

HSP-SENSITIVITY TRAINING TECHNIQUE NO. 1

YOUR ONENESS WITH MIND

Sit down in your chair, relax, breathe deeply, and let a feeling of peace envelop your mind. In the silence, ask yourself the question, "What lies behind the door of mind?" Repeat the question three times, emphasizing first the word *what,* then the words *lies behind,* and third the words *the door of mind.* In this manner silently inquire, *"What* lies behind the door of mind? What *lies behind* the door of mind? What lies behind *the door of mind?"*

Now visualize in your mind's eye a large door. The panel is ornately carved of dark, lustrous wood. See the door grow in size before you as you mentally move toward it. It becomes larger and larger until it seems to reach into the infinite. You notice, now, that three words emerge from the intricate design carved into the wood. The words glowing a. misty white, read: *DOOR OF MIND.* Keep your vision focused upon these words until they become large and distinct. Mentally continue to walk toward the panel.

You note, now, that the door is beginning to swing open; shafts of golden light are streaming through it. As you proceed in your imagination to walk through the door, a beautiful garden comes into view. It is the garden of the world.

A winding path leads into the garden. You begin striding along that path. You see the roses banked along each side. You smell the fragrance. The grass is green and soft. Your ears catch the buzzing of bees as they sip the sweet nectar of the flowers. The melodious singing of the birds greets you as well as the chattering of a squirrel as it scurries through the garden.

As you proceed along the path, you note the beauty of each flower, each blade of grass, each expression of life. You feel yourself to be *one* with this life—one with everything that lives—one with universal Mind.

The path winds along a wooded glen circling a placid lake. As you come to the lake, you see a finger of land that reaches out into the water. You walk out upon that point of land, enjoying the calm serenity of the water that stretches before you.

You stop and look down into the crystal water and observe the reflection of a cloud that is drifting overhead. Gradually you lift your eyes into the heavens and behold the same cloud as it moves across the sky. With the eyes of imagination you follow the cloud until it is but a small silvery point of light in the vastness of the sky, and then it is gone.

In the silence, now, you feel yourself to be one with this vastness. You are one with the universe. You pause now and in silence affirm this oneness. You declare of yourself, *"I am one with all life. I am one with the infinite reaches of Mind. I am one with all power, with all love, with all beauty, and with all that life is. In the silent depths of me, I know this is true."* (Capture and sustain in quietness, now, the *oneness* your trip has brought you.) After a period of deep contemplation, conclude:

And so it is!

SUMMARY CAPSULES

YOU, THE UNSEEN TENANT IN THE HOUSE-OF-SELF

Back of the facade of appearance—back of your physical image—dwells a mysterious and unseen tenant. It is the Real You. It is *mysterious* because you know it so slightly as yet. It is *unseen* for the mental you is invisible, the invisible essence living within the physical House-of-Self (body). To probe the nature of this unseen self is the object of the Science of Higher Sense Perception.

YOUR PSI-ABILITY AWAITS YOUR USE

The Real You has a vast scale of ability, ranging from sense-powers at the lower end to psi-powers at the upper end. Psi-ability is the behind-the-scene force that underlies your higher-sensory potentials of telepathy, clairvoyance, clairaudience, retrocognition, precognition, intuition, etc. You can learn to tap psi-ability to demonstrate guidance, protection, wisdom, financial success, and personal achievement.

YOU ARE ONE WITH INFINITE MIND

As the ocean *waves,* so the universe *peoples.* The universal principle of mind, pushing itself forth into expression, manifests as you and your fellowman. As the wave cannot be separate from the ocean, you cannot be separate from infinite Mind. Likewise, as the depths of the wave extend down into the potential of the sea, so your powers extend into the depths of Mind.

YOU ARE SOMETHING BIGGER THAN YOU DREAM

Something does not come out of nothing. How can you be a knower without a *source* of knowingness from which to come? How can you be creative without a *cause* of creativity from which to come? Man must infer the existence of *Something* that makes his knowing, his creativity, his love, and his aspirations possible. He cannot deny Something bigger than himself.

YOUR RIGHT TO HSP POTENTIALITIES

Thou hast made him to have dominion over the earth and hast put all things under his feet. It is written that man, apex of the evolutionary process, has been endowed with *all things*—all powers, all abilities, all potentialities. These powers are your natural right. They are not abnormal but normal, normal for you when you develop your *higher* sense perception.

2

How to Demonstrate Radiant
Health and Happiness

Aileen's face was aglow. "Look," she exclaimed, "I can walk! I can walk!" Then somewhat thoughtfully, as though savoring a miracle, she repeated, "I can walk without help."

Standing before me was Aileen M., a lady in her early fifties, the picture of radiant health.

The happiness that shone from her eyes made her appear more lovely than I had ever seen her. She was walking on cloud nine. The miracle was that she was walking at all!

I remembered the day, seven months earlier, when the phone rang and a friend of Aileen's asked me if I would visit her in the hospital. The friend told me that Aileen was not expected to live through the weekend. This was on a Thursday.

That afternoon I went to the hospital. As I walked into the room, there was no movement or recognition from the lady whose quiet form lay in the bed. Aileen was in an almost totally paralytic condition. As I took her hand and told her who I was, there was only a slight response.

I talked with her, leading her in meditation, knowing that although there was little conscious recognition, my words would register at an interior level.

The following day I returned, and the next, and the next. So through the weeks and months, we talked and meditated together. With each visit, there was a growing response and a greater freedom of physical movement. The day arrived when Aileen left the hospital and, with the aid of a walker, regained complete normalcy.

How resentment blocks the flow of life

During the sessions with Aileen at the hospital, I found in her a deep resentment that had blocked the free flow of life and contributed to her paralysis.

She harbored a deep-seated resentment toward her husband who had recently passed on leaving affairs in an impossible state of disarray. Her resentment over the estate had grown to a frenzied pitch. "If only he were still around," her thoughts about her husband ran, "I'd tell him what a mess he made of things and how inconsiderate he was to leave me like this!" But, he was beyond the lashing of her tongue, and she had locked her resentment tightly inside her.

Coupled with her distress and frustration was a feeling of guilt for her present attitude toward her husband. After all, he was the person with whom she had spent over thirty years of her life! She condemned him while knowing full well that criticism is ungracious. On top of it all, Aileen resented the black clothes of mourning that her friends had expected her to wear.

Suddenly, she was hit by a strange paralysis that puzzled her medical advisors. They could find no physical origin for the crippling illness that was threatening her very life. This is when Aileen's friend called me.

The principles involved in meta-healing

During the months of her recovery, Aileen and I talked of health and how meta-thinking (higher thinking) can be used to demonstrate a state of wholeness.

One day I mentioned the story of the man with the large block of granite who told a friend that he was going to sculpture it into an elephant.

"But," responded his friend, "this seems like an impossible task!"

"Not at all," replied the sculptor. "All I have to do is chip away everything that isn't an elephant!"

"It is like this with health," I explained to Aileen. "All you must do to achieve health is to eliminate everything that isn't health. You must eliminate resentment, worry, disgust, condemnation, fear, hatred, guilt and all unlovely elements that block a radiant image. It is not a matter of making health real, but of removing the unreal. This is meta-healing."

The *real* is the radiant, balanced, pulsating, vitalizing, animating essence that forms the base of all life. It is the life principle, the COSMIC RADIANT. This *cosmic radiant* expresses as the vitality and incessancy of cell division. It expresses as the animation and intelligence of the maturation process. It expresses as the balance and orderliness of the life cycle. Indeed, it expresses as the vibrant beauty of the atom itself!

Everywhere you look, you see the cosmic radiant—the life principle—expressing in all its perfection (unless man has blocked it or polluted it or corrupted it).

This is what Aileen came to understand. When you are in tune with the cosmic radiant, you experience that which is natural to it—health, happiness, and the joys of being. When you think off-key, you force yourself into a state of discord and disease (*dis*-ease). You constrict your psi-abilities. You are out-of-tune with the Infinite.

What Aileen learned to do was to chip away everything that was not health and happiness. She chipped away the unwanted stone of resentment until a statue of forgiveness was all that was left. She came to realize that when you are out-of-tune with the *real* you experience a degree of paralysis in some area. It may be the area of business, financial failure, personality problems, frigidity, health problems, unhappiness, or the like—somewhere the flow of good will be blocked.

If you are experiencing a state of health or happiness that is something less than desired, learn to raise the tone of your thinking. Learn to think on-key and put yourself in tune with the COSMIC RADIANT of livingness, vitality, energy, order, and beauty within you now. *Remove the unreal and let the real express* with the following Psi-Programming Pointer.

Ψ   Psi-Programming Pointer

I PUT MYSELF IN TUNE WITH THE "COSMIC RADIANT" BY KEEPING MY THOUGHTS ON A POSITIVE, HARMONI-OUS KEY. I LET GO OF NARROW, PARALYZING, CON-STRICTING IMAGES AND LET A NEW RADIANCE ANIMATE ME.

Awareness of the COSMIC RADIANT

Aileen's patience in attuning herself to the cosmic radiant paid off. She rose triumphantly above the resentment that had wrecked her health and happiness.

It was during the time I was counseling with her that my own awareness of the cosmic radiant was dramatically highlighted, demonstrating to me that this radiant principle of life can be seen visually during moments of expanded consciousness.

The place was the desert outside Phoenix and the month was July. The day was warm but not uncomfortable. I was lecturing in Phoenix that summer and, following a talk that I had given one Sunday morning, my wife and I drove out in the desert for a picnic.

I can recall the experience as if it were yesterday. Leaving the car, we hiked to a view-spot by a giant saguaro cactus. Here we enjoyed our lunch and were revelling in the vast, quiet beauty of the scene before us when I became aware that the colors were more exciting than they had ever been to me before.

I remarked to my wife about the unusual beauty of the hills. We were both caught up in the excitement of the day and in the grandeur around us, but for me it was truly an unusual vista. Whether my wife saw the colors I saw, I cannot be sure. I only know that for me it was an exciting experience in consciousness!

The colors I saw were intense. There were hues of gold shading off into orange, pale blues, and purples, with dazzling combinations *all* joined together in what may be described as a visual symphony! It was as if the universe were one vibrant, radiant, harmonious, cosmic whole.

There was no abrupt beginning nor end to my intensified perception of the colors. It was more of a stepping up in consciousness as my appreciation grew and then a toning down in color intensity. Through it all I felt a sense of oneness with the scene before me.

The new world of meta-powers

Many people have similar experiences of expanded awareness when they see or hear or feel the cosmic radiant of life. Thinking back, you may be able to remember an instance when you enjoyed a heightened sense of awareness—when the charm of a landscape, the splendor of a sunrise or sunset, or the beauty of a loved one's face took on added intensity and significance. With the use of the techniques set out in this book, these experiences will tend to be more frequent and exciting for you.

One of the basic premises of the Science of Higher Sense Perception is that the world you see is but the *beginning of vision.* The world you hear is but the *beginning of sound.* There is more to be seen, heard, and experienced than you have ever dreamed. There are vast reaches beyond your present level of awareness which, when you glimpse them, will make you realize that the past has brought you only to the starting gate of perception.

There is a range of colors that you have never seen. There are levels of sound that your ear has never heard. There is a sensation of health and wholeness that you have never felt. There are extended powers of mind waiting to be tapped by you. *There is a higher-sense-perception world beyond the world you know!*

The term *meta* may be used to describe such higher sensory experiences. *Meta* is defined by the dictionary as that which is *"behind or beyond; more comprehensive than; transcending."* In the pages that follow, you will be introduced to techniques of meta-healing, meta-hearing, meta-seeing, and other manifestations of higher sense perception.

One of the outstanding exponents of the larger self, Rudolph Steiner, in *Knowledge of the Higher Worlds,* says, "When passing through a beautiful mountain district, the traveller with a depth of soul and wealth of feeling has different experiences from one who is poor in feeling. Only what we experience within ourselves unlocks for us the beauties of the outer world."[1]

It is the purpose of the Science of Higher Sense Perception to help you cultivate the interior consciousness and wealth of feeling of which Steiner writes, leading you to a *knowledge* of higher worlds—a new world of meta-powers.

Enhance life by observing from a higher inner place

The *height* of the interior place from which you view your world determines how *far* you can see mentally. Natural science has led man to the ends of the world, physically speaking, but the inner world which gives meaning to the outer remains for the most part unexplored.

That unexplored inner world is more pertinent to the outer than is generally realized. It was with Jeans, Eddington, and (h scientific thinkers that the connection between the two worlds first became clear. They advanced the concept that *there is both a world to be observed and an observer to behold it.* Moreover, *the observed world cannot be divorced from the observer.* In other words, you cannot say that *here* is the one who sees and over *here* is what is seen. What you see and hear and feel, depend upon where you are. Not where you are physically but *mentally,* for it is the mind that sees and hears—not the eye and ear.

Hence, the outer view of life that you see depends upon the inner place *where you are* in consciousness. As Steiner sugge ts, the observer with a wealth of feeling will see grandeur in a mountain view which is non-existent for the person poor in consciousness. The observed cannot be divorced from the observer. Thus, the way to enhance that which is observed is for the observer to climb to a greater height—a meta-height, a height above and beyond that already known.

The way to achieve a "wealth of feeling"

Why are some *poor in consciousness* while others enjoy a *wealth of feeling?* Consider it this way: you are the awakening of life as

---

[1]Steiner, Rudolf, *Knowledge of the Higher Worlds and its Attainment.* London: Rudolf Steiner Publishing Co., 1937, p. 21.

personalized being. This awakening occurs as you respond to the challenges of life and results in varying levels or degrees of consciousness. Within you there is the possibility of a greater awakening, for every day is an adventure that bids you awaken and develop a perception that is more acute. Each level of awareness that you attain forms a rung from which you may step up to a more advanced state of perception.

You might think of consciousness as a ladder, with the distance between each rung representing families of living things. As the ladder stretches upward, there is the rung of rudimentary consciousness (plant), simple consciousness (animal), self-consciousness (man), and superconsciousness (the real Self.)

Man is standing upon a rung that is well up on the ladder of life, but there is no reason for thinking that the ladder stops with man *as he appears today.* Above the rung upon which he now stands are other rungs he can reach as he extends the five senses he now has and dev l ɔs expanded sensory percep ɪon.

Hence, the way to achieve a wealth of feeling, the way to climb to a higer ru ɪg of consciousness, is to accelerate your own mental unfoldment. This you will be doing as you apply the HSP Sensitivity Training Techniques in the chapters that follow.

From sense reception to higher sensory perception

The first step in accelerating your mental unfoldment is to understand how your present faculties developed. In the upward push of the principle of life into form, certain sense receptors developed, enabling the individual *life expression* to adjust successfully to its environment. In the higher organisms, including man, specific sense organs (receptors) developed, permitting a fairly accurate reception of a wide variety of complex stimuli such as sights, smells, tastes, sounds, heat, cold, etc.

Have you ever wondered as to the origin of such receptors? Did the eye come first and then the ability to see? Or, did the sense of sight come first and then the eye? What is the source from which this ability comes? What enables the development of such sense equipment? And, what further *extended* receptors await unfoldment?

For example, it is a known fact that powers observed in man exist in rudimentary form far down the ladder of life. Protoplasm, the basic unit of all living matter, possesses a characteristic excitability. The amoeba, a unicellular organism, is excitable in a vague way. In man, the ability to experience excitement is highly specialized.

In the forward thrust of life, that which exists potentially at simpler levels becomes differentiated in highly specialized sense receptors as the form evolves. Through the specialized receptors you now have, you experience the sensations of seeing, hearing, feeling, tasting, and smelling. But are not these senses, in themselves, the rudimentary form of still higher senses?

What is the source from which the five senses come? If they spring from a principle, cannot a higher use of that principle be made? In *The Great Chain of Life,* Joseph Wood Krutch says:

> Animals, so it seems, did not learn to see because they developed what we call an eye. On the contrary, they developed eyes because they were already able, in some sense, to see. And this ability to see is not in any way explained or accounted for by the fullest understanding of the optical principles involved in the highly developed eye itself.[2]

And, as Dr. Gustav Stromberg in *The Soul of the Universe* explains:

> Our sensations and other mental attributes are not by-products of atomic configurations in each individual brain; they have a cosmic foundation and ultimate origin common to all individuals.[3]

Krutch and Stromberg's statements suggest that vision resides in a principle of sight that is everywhere present. If sight is limited, it is not the fault of the principle but of the equipment through which the principle must operate. The same would be true of the principle of hearing, and feeling, and sensing.

Likewise, health abides in a principle of wholeness that is present here and now. If health is restricted, it is not the fault of the principle but of the consciousness through which the principle must express.

-----

[2]Krutch, Joseph Wood, *The Great Chain of Life.* Boston: Houghton Mifflin Co., 1956, p. 8.

[3] Stromberg, Gustav, *The Soul of The Universe.* Los Angeles: Educational Research Institute, 1940., p. 168.

The case of Cayce's astonishing psi-equipment

A remarkable man whose equipment was anything but limited was Edgar Cayce. His remarkable powers attest to the fact that the faculty of vision is greater than the sense of sight functioning through the human eye. He had the faculty of meta-vision—a *higher* vision that saw beyond the limitations of sense perception.

Cayce developed a phenomenal technique for using his extended vision in humanitarian work at a clinic in Virginia. He discovered that while in a subconscious state he was able to *see* the cause behind physical, mental and emotional problems people brought to him. His diagnostic accuracy was startling.

Gina Cerminara, the author of *Many Mansions* (a research study of Cayce's method), tells how Cayce would lie down, place himself in a self-induced hypnotic trance, and dictate to a secretary his diagnoses. Frequently, requests came from people at great distances from Virginia, people he never met.

Speaking of one case, the author relates:

> One of the most dramatic examples of the manner in which Cayce's hypnotic clairvoyance demonstrated itself is to be seen in the case of a young girl in Selma, Alabama, who unaccountably lost her reason and was committed to a mental institution. Her brother, deeply concerned, requested Cayce's help. Cayce lay down on his couch, took a few deep breaths, and put himself to sleep. He then accepted a brief hypnotic suggestion that he *see* and diagnose the body of the girl in question. After a pause of a few moments he began to speak, as all hypnotic subjects will when so instructed. Unlike most hypnotic subjects, however, he began to outline, as if possessed of X-ray vision, the physical condition of the demented girl.[4]

Following the diagnosis by Edgar Cayce, the treatment he suggested was undertaken and the girl was restored to normalcy.

Cayce found a way to effectively use the principles of vision independent of the sense of sight, proving that the principle is only as limited as the equipment through which it must function.

---

[4]Cerminara, Gina, *Many Mansions.* New York: William Morrow & Co., Inc. Publishers, 1953, p. 12.

How to unlock your limited sensory equipment

If the eye developed because man was already able, in some sense, to see, then there is a *principle* of sight. Left alone, that principle is capable of evolving finer modes of expression through refinement, adaptation, mutation, natural selection, etc. In time, Krutch's *ability to see* inevitably would develop higher means by which to express in man—means such as telepathy and clairvoyance.

However, why wait? Why not unlock your limited sensory equipment now and add to it *expanded powers of seeing, hearing, feeling, and perceiving?* Just as your five senses evolved from rudimentary forms inherent in primitive life, those senses are the rudimentary forms of expanded powers awaiting your development now.

For example, it might be said that sensing is a rudimentary forerunner of perception.

A dictionary gives this definition of *perception: "Awareness of the elements of environment through physical sensation—color, etc; physical sensation interpreted in the light of experience; direct or intuitive cognition; insight; a capacity for comprehension."*

Perception is superior to the five senses, for perception is what gives meaning to that which you sense. As a great one of long ago said, "Having eyes to see they see not, and having ears to hear they hear not." Without perception your sensory equipment is limited. Often you see without understanding and hear without comprehension.

Perception is an extension of *sensing.* It is what man must develop if he is to unlock the potentialities within his mind and use his faculties wisely, effectively, and successfully.

The woman who wished she wasn't psychic

Of the many people whom I counsel, a large number have had psychic experiences for which they seek explanations. Such was the case with the lady who sat across the desk from me one morning—Carolyn Y. She was a woman in her late forties. As we talked, she seemed mentally normal, but nervous and depressed.

She explained that she had been plagued with a health problem as well as a psychic susceptibility that marred her happiness.

I asked Carolyn to tell me the nature of her psychic experiences. She mentioned a number of fragmentary ones that were not too dramatic. Then, she related one that had both frightened and astonished her.

"It was on the farm when I was just entering the teen years of life," she related. "I was standing in the kitchen of our home. My mother had gone to the bedroom to rest. My father, brother, and Jim, a hired man, were cutting trees over the hill which was back of the house and some distance away. As I stood looking out the window, suddenly the scene changed. I was no longer seeing the normal view from the window. I could see *over* the hill!

"I found myself witnessing an accident. The wagon my father was in had overturned and he was pinned beneath a wheel. I saw the face of my father clearly, just as clearly as I now see you. His face was writhed in pain, and then it became still and white. I felt that my father had died.

"At this moment my mother, who had awakened quite suddenly from her nap, came into the kitchen. The vision was gone, but I told her what I had seen. We both knew that something was wrong.

"We were still wondering what we should do and trying unsuccessfully to convince ourselves that what I had seen was nonsense, when we heard voices at the back door. It was my brother and Jim carrying my father. He was not dead, but he'd had an accident. His left leg was badly crushed. As my brother and Jim told us of the mishap, every detail agreed with the accident I had described to Mother. I had seen something that was impossible with normal sight.

"Through the years I've been very sensitive psychically," continued Carolyn. "I have had many other experiences like this which I have learned to keep to myself. I'm only telling you now for you are someone who understands.

"The thing is," Carolyn confided, "that this ability, whatever it is, has brought me nothing but distress. Other people think it's strange. So, I find myself hiding it and feeling guilty about it. Frankly, I wish I didn't have it!"

"Carolyn, you must never feel ashamed of having clairvoyant ability. Don't try to repress it or hide it or deny it! What you have will some day be the norm. Don't think of yourself as being abnormal. Clairvoyance is perfectly normal to an expanded consciousness."

I suggested to Carolyn that she approach her ability as a positive asset, learning to use it according to the sound and safe principles of HSP training.

We talked about the principles behind higher sensory perception—that the five senses are but rudimentary forms of what mankind will one day enjoy; that the eye developed because man was already able to see; that the ear developed because man was already able to hear; that clairvoyance, telepathy and other extended faculties will be the norm for man when he comes to accept higher sense perception as normal.

How negative thoughts bring physical ills

"Why, just recently," I told Carolyn, "the press carried a report of an eminent scientist who predicts that among the developments the future holds for man is communication between people on a telepathic level rather than verbal."

"Do you really think," Carolyn asked, "that people will be able to give up their ceaseless yakking?"

"Not without a struggle," I admitted, "but I, too, believe that normal progress for man is toward telepathic communication. In addition, one day it will be *normal* to use meta-healing to eliminate the root of emotionally-induced illness. It will be *normal* to demonstrate guidance through clairvoyance. It will be *normal* to use directed-dream power for creative insight. In fact, it is normal right now for those who have extended their sensory equipment to receive HSP stimuli."

Man's sensory equipment is like a television set. If your television is not built to pick up color impulses or if certain channels are beyond your range of reception, the waves emitted by the broadcasting studio will not be received by your set and will, therefore, go unenjoyed. Yet, it is perfectly normal to get color reception on *some* sets; *some* sets will be getting the channels you cannot reach!

So it is with the reception of HSP "channels." *Some* who are receptive to higher sense impulses will pick up telepathic and clairvoyant "waves" emitted by "broadcasting" minds. For *others,* however, whose mental equipment is not yet expanded, HSP impulses will go unused.

"Carolyn," I said, "you are one of those people who is already receptive to HSP *broadcasting.* It is evidence of a superior potential. Don't apologize for it or feel guilty about being different."

"If it's so superior," Carolyn replied, "why can't I use it some way to demonstrate health. Health is what I really want!"

"Maybe it's because you have never tried using it for that," I suggested. "In fact, your resentment over a power that makes you appear strange in other's eyes, your guilt over it, and your negative reactions toward it are enough to make you sick!"

Carolyn listened attentively.

"What you need to do," I explained, "is to use your sensitiveness *constructively* instead of *negatively.* You see, meta-thinking can help you demonstrate a state of health. Meta-thinking means higher thinking. It means replacing negative elements of self-guilt, resentment, shame, regret, and the like, with positive elements of self-confidence, poise, self-respect, inner dignity, and faith. This is meta-healing."

"Positive thinking," I continued, "is learning to think on-key. It puts you in tune with the universal principle of life. I think of that principle as the COSMIC RADIANT, for it is the radiant livingness, vitality, energy, order, and beauty inherent in all animated beings. With your psi-sensitiveness, Carolyn, you should be able to sense that cosmic radiant and attune yourself to it!"

I gave this lady, *who wished she wasn't psychic,* a Psi-Programming Pointer like the one that follows. As she used it and we worked together, her nervousness disappeared and she became poised and confident. Best of all, she transformed her psi-ability from a nuisance into a useful tool. She used it to lift her consciousness to a level where health and happiness manifested!

Psi-Programming Pointer
I NOW ATTUNE MY THOUGHTS TO A HIGH OCTAVE
WHERE HEALTH, HARMONY, AND HAPPINESS ARE NOR-
MAL. I KEEP MY THINKING ON-KEY BY REPLACING NEG-
ATIVE IMAGES WITH THOUGHTS OF POSITIVE TONE.

A man who lived on "high"

Are you seeing health? Are you seeing life as joy and fulfillment? If the principle of vision sees independently of the limited
instrument, *isn't it reasonable* that by lifting your sight to a vision
of wholeness, higher octaves on the scale of health may be
demonstrated?

It is! For health is tuning to a higher frequency, a frequency of
wholeness. It is putting oneself in tune with the Infinite. This is
what Clifford A. did.

Cliff, a member of one of my classes, was a fascinating person.
He was a man who grasped HSP principles immediately.

"Why," he said, after the first class session together, "this is
what I have always felt was true. This is it!"

Cliff laughed a great deal, and when he wasn't laughing, he was
smiling. He said to me, "Have you ever heard of anyone who
couldn't get mad? Well, people think this is strange. But, I just
don't get mad."

While waiting for my reaction, he continued, "I find life too
exciting and too wonderful to spend even a small amount of it in
being angry or in holding grudges or in criticizing people."

Cliff's attitude delighted me. Here was a person who had
already grasped the concept of living on a high octave—of living in
tune with the cosmic radiant. He *was* radiant! He was the picture
of health. His personality sparkled.

"Cliff," I said jokingly, "you don't seem to have a trouble in
the world."

"I don't," he replied.

I could believe him!

Sometimes a person has to work very diligently to demonstrate
a feeling of *oneness with life.* Sometimes he must practice over

and over again the training techniques that lead to expanded sense perception. Cliff was one of those fortunate people who grasps the principles instantly.

Finding a science that taught a way-of-life which he already endorsed was more than he had ever dreamed. He was ecstatic about it. He quickly found himself in love with life and living from the cosmic radiant.

"Cliff," I remarked one evening when he seemed especially exuberant, "I hope you're not on drugs!"

"Who needs drugs? With the belt this philosophy gives me," he said, "I can get high on water!" And he laughed one of those very contagious laughs that exclaims in loud, clear tones— *"Life is wonderful!"*

Health and happiness are your heritage

Life *is* wonderful! And, health is *natural* to it. Happiness is *natural* to it. The person who does not enjoy health and happiness has somehow struck a mental chord that is out of tune with the Infinite. For some reason he is functioning on a negative frequency that puts him out of touch with what is REAL. He then experiences some degree of limitation, constriction, paralysis, distress, or *dis*-ease.

Remember what Aileen had to do? She had to chip away that which was UNREAL. She had to discard resentment, criticism, self-guilt, condemnation, and regret and substitute positive qualities. By doing so, she reached the REAL; she reached the level of the cosmic radiant.

What can you do to bring your thinking up to this level and experience, as Cliff did, the glorious realization that life is wonderful? Just this . . . you can practice meta-thinking (higher thinking).

Here are the positive thought-qualities that raise you to the frequency of the cosmic radiant. Notice that they spell the word H-E-A-L-T-H. They are qualities which those who enjoy the fullness of health and happiness seem to have in common. Cultivate them and you will be putting yourself in tune with the principle of life (the COSMIC RADIANT).

HAPPINESS—To make a little happiness happen each day is the best tonic there is. As the writer of *Proverbs* said centuries ago, "A merry heart doeth good like a medicine."

ENTHUSIASM—To have enthusiasm for life is to radiate a special delight (inner light) which makes plans and ideas come alive. It is to be *"en theos"* or *inspired* by the *superconscious mind* within you.

APPRECIATION—To appreciate is to find that which is worthy of praise within yourself and within those around you. It is to replace criticism, condemnation, and resentment with recognition of a basic good inherent in everything.

LOVE—To practice love is to give joyously for the joy of giving and to forgive freely. It is the ability to love people for what they are, if not for what they do.

TRANQUILITY—To live in tranquility is to banish all that would make you hurried, worried, and tense. It gives you a poise that takes the pressure out of living.

HARMONY—To harvest harmony is to do the little extra things that keep peace and bring friendliness, cooperation, consideration, order, and joy into your relationship with others.

As you practice these positive mental qualities, you will raise the tone of your consciousness and demonstrate meta-healing. However, the results are not restricted to health; they include happiness as well.

Now, make these attitudes doubly effective by using the following HSP Sensitivity Training Technique which will help you to:

Have Happiness

Endorse Enthusiasm

Affirm Appreciation

Love Life

Think Tranquility

Harvest Harmony

The first sensitivity training technique you practiced at the end of Chapter One was designed to bring you a feeling of *oneness* with the universe. Now, use the following training to develop your sensitivity to the *radiant principle of livingness* latent within you. Remember, this training is to be an experience in consciousness *as* you practice it. Enter into it with *feeling* and *sincerity*.

HOW TO PREPARE FOR THE TRAINING

First, make arrangements to prevent interruption during your training period.

Second, seat yourself comfortably in the chair you have selected for your psi-sensitivity training. Why the same chair each time? So that you will associate it with your training periods and the very act of sitting in it will prepare you psychologically for another session. Each time you enter your *consciousness training,* you will find yourself slipping into it more quickly and deeply.

Third, quietly read the following consciousness-expanding exercise. Read it two or three times, until you can repeat the essence of it mentally with your eyes closed. At the end, pause in absolute silence and *feel* the *significance* of what your *oneness with the radiant principle of life* really means.

HSP-SENSITIVITY TRAINING TECHNIQUE NO. 2

ATTUNING TO THE COSMIC RADIANT

You are seated in your chair. Relax, breathe deeply, and enter the calm of your deeper self. Now, in your mind's eye, you behold a large, richly carved door with the words emblazoned in misty white, *DOOR OF MIND.*

Feel yourself arising now from your chair and moving toward this door. As you do so, it swings wide open revealing a scene of magnificent beauty and distant snow-covered mountains. You see yourself mentally walking through the door and winding your way along a flower-lined path. The path leads you to the shore of a serene lake. You remember, now, being here before. You remember following a cloud in your imagination until it blended with infinity and gave you the feeling that your own being blended with the universe in a realization of oneness.

This time as you reach that feeling of oneness, the setting sun hits the cloud which your eye is following and turns it a shimmering, radiant white. The edge of the cloud is ringed with silver. As it glides through the deep azure sky, it somehow comes alive.

Your eye follows it to the dark horizon, and, as the sun sets, the stars appear one by one. You become aware of the vast cosmic order and balance that holds the stars in place. You actually seem to hear the harmony of the spheres.

In the hush and awe of the moment, you become aware of a presence you have never felt before. From the tiniest cell to the largest star, each thing seems animated—animated with an energy, a vigor, a vibration, a harmony, a radiance that constitutes its very being. This universal radiance—this principle of livingness—is the COSMIC RADIANT!

You now acclaim the presence of this same cosmic radiant within yourself. You raise the frequency of your thought to that on which the cosmic radiant vibrates, and life, vitality, and health surge through your being.

You now make yourself an heir to HAPPINESS by endorsing ENTHUSIASM. You affirm an attitude of APPRECIATION and do that which proves your LOVE of life. You bring peace to your heart as you think TRANQUILITY and harvest HARMONY.

Your thoughts are tuned to a cosmic pitch, and you feel the presence of life's animating radiance within you. Your body is aglow with a new vitality that courses through it now. That which is unreal drops away and only the REAL is left.

You say to yourself now, *"Every cell of my being is attuned to the Infinite. It vibrates on the same key as the cosmic life principle. Health and happiness are mine!"*

You rest and relax, now, abiding in the consciousness of attunement you have created. (Close your eyes after reading the above consciousness-expanding exercise several times, and put yourself through the steps it suggests.) Then, let a feeling of deep silence pervade your being. Sustain yourself in that silence until you can truly say:

And so it is!

SUMMARY CAPSULES

WHEN NEW WINDOWS OF HSP ARE OPENED

There are five main windows through which you behold the world—hearing, feeling, tasting, smelling, and seeing. These windows relate you to your outer environment. If those windows were to be enlarged and expanded, imagine how much more of the world you would be able to perceive. Imagine, too, the possibility of discovering mystery windows you never opened before—windows of HSP that bring an *expanded* world into view!

WHERE THE SENSES SEEM TO END, HSP BEGINS

Although the range of man's physical senses is limited, the principle that underlies those senses is limitless. In other words, the creative principle is greater than its creations. The eye is but the beginning of vision. The ear is but the beginning of hearing. Beyond the eye and ear, HSP begins! Its range is boundless and will unfold for you as you make yourself a better instrument through which the creative principle can function.

WHAT META-HEALING CAN DO FOR YOU

As you expand your awareness and begin to expect more of yourself, you will discover new facets of personal power. One of these is the power to align yourself with the universal principle of life and experience its healing power. This is meta-healing. The *principle of life* is a throbbing, pulsating, vibrant, animate presence—the Cosmic Radiant. When you are in tune with it, there can be no discord, no *dis*-ease, within you.

HOW ILLNESS AND UNHAPPINESS DISAPPEAR

The cause of health and happiness problems may lie in something *present* in consciousness or something *absent* from consciousness. For example, constriction of health may be due to the *presence* of resentment, distrust, antagonism, self-guilt, etc. Or it may be due to the *absence* of love, harmony, forgiveness, etc. Regardless, the state of illness or unhappiness will disappear to the extent that you think on-key and replace discordant, negative thoughts with positive ones.

WHERE YOU NOW STAND ON THE LADDER

The daily conditions you experience belong to the rung of the ladder upon which you now stand. Your consciousness-level externalizes a place for you that is equal to your state of mind—be it happiness or unhappiness. If your consciousness is discordant, it cannot produce the music of health and happiness; if it is harmonious, it cannot produce unhappiness. Begin where you stand now and step up to meta-thinking, meta-healing, and happiness.

3

How to Develop the Higher
Sense of Metavision

It was back in the early mining-fever days of the West. A young man, a graduate of Colorado School of Mines, accepted an engineering job in Nevada. With his wife and a tiny daughter, he moved to the budding boom town of Goldfield.

This young engineer, whom I shall call Mark A., built a small cottage for his family in the residential area (three isolated houses in all) at the far end of town. The mine and mill where he worked were several miles distant on the desert.

One night, while on the graveyard shift, Mark was riding a lift to a lower level when the hoist chain broke and cut a deep gash in his scalp. He fell fifteen feet to the mill floor and lay there unconscious until a fellow worker found him. The man left his lantern by Mark's side and ran for help.

Mark, while alone, partly regained consciousness. His one thought was, "I must get home." Dazed, he pulled himself to his feet and picked up the lantern. His steps were unsure, but the thought, "I *must* get home," kept him moving. He had not gone more than half a mile on his painful trek across the desert waste when his lantern went out.

Meanwhile, his wife, who was asleep, awakened with a strange feeling that something was wrong. She did not know what the cause for her apprehension was, but she sensed that her husband needed her and was trying to get to her.

Without an objective reason for doing so, Mark's wife hurried to the front room and awakened her tiny daughter, whose bed was the livingroom couch. "Quickly," she said to the little girl, "go get into my bed. Daddy's coming home, and they will need the couch for him."

Then, Mark's wife went to the window, pinned back the lace curtains, and placed a lighted lamp close to the pane. It was just as if she could *see* her husband wandering lost in the blackness of the desert night.

After what seemed an eternity, the young wife heard a sound at the door. She opened it. Mark, more dead than alive, fell exhausted into the room. He had seen her lamp in the window; it was the beacon that guided his staggering steps homeward. Without it, he could have wandered until he collapsed and died in the desert darkness.

Mark's wife was hurrying for bandages and water to bathe his head when she heard a second knock at the door. It was the men from the mill. They had come to tell the young wife about the accident and the horrible news that Mark could not be found. To their astonishment, they saw him on the floor of the cottage. They helped lift him onto the couch and sent for medical aid. Mark recovered and went on to become an outstanding mining engineer.

Acting upon instances of guidance and warning

Mark's story was one I told to some of my HSP class members one evening. I finished it with the conclusion, "The higher-sense-perception message Mark's wife received saved his life—saved it because she *acted* upon that message."

Dwight, one of the members, remarked, "It's just great, of course, when people are intuitive like that, but I've never had any HSP impressions."

"Dwight," I replied, "you have the equipment to get higher-sensory messages. Everyone has! And I *know* that you've experienced this higher sense faculty whether you're aware of it or not."

My listener did not seem convinced, so I continued.

"HSP guidance can come in many forms; it may be gentle or dramatic. It can express as a mild degree of uneasiness—a slight recognition that something is wrong. (This is the kind it's easy to ignore.) It can come as a more insistent sensing or seeing that may motivate a person to action, as was the case with the young wife who sensed the desperate need of her husband and put a light in the window."

If you happen to feel as Dwight did—that you have had no higher sensory experiences—look back over your life. Examine it, and you will remember instances when you had a gentle feeling or hunch you should have heeded. Very likely, you have remarked at some time, "I had a *feeling* I should have gone." Or, "I could *see* that something was wrong."

It does not matter the name you use in describing this subtle guidance—hunch, clairvoyance, premonition—everyone has the equipment to receive it. Just receiving it, of course, is not enough. Like Mark's wife, you must *act* upon it if guidance and right action are to result.

I do not imply that you should follow every subjective whim that clamors for attention, but an intuitive urge that is truly the operation of *higher sense perception* can be trusted.

It was Dwight speaking again: "How do I recognize an urge that can be trusted? In fact, how do I become sensitive enough to get an HSP message in the first place?"

"You use the psi-programming techniques I have for you," I replied. "But, first, let's understand the principle behind such messages—the principle of non-objective communication—and what it can do for you."

Probing the principle of non-objective communication

Mark could not have communicated with his wife—indeed, Dwight could not have talked with me—if there were not an underlying principle of communication in the universe.

In the world of invention, man uses this principle in many objective forms—the intercom, walkie-talkie, telephone, telegraph, radio, television, radar, sonar, telestar, and the like. Man has managed to perform communication miracles. His voice can span the oceans and interstellar space to the Moon.

He has managed this feat because behind the devices his imagination has created is a principle which makes those creations possible. Telephone, television, and other such means of communication are but objective copies of non-objective communicative means that exist in the great untapped potential of universal Mind.

For virtually every objective invention, there is a similar non-objective counterpart. The telephone echoes the telepathic principle resident in universal Mind. Television reflects principles inherent in clairvoyance and clairaudience. The original sending and receiving device is not the radio or short-wave set. It is the non-objective mental equipment within each living thing.

No matter where you probe, you can see a communication principle at work. Take the inanimate level for example: there is a cohesiveness or communicativeness evident in molecular attraction.

On the level of single-celled life, there is cooperation and communication. The loose community of cells that live together and form the aquatic man-of-war beautifully illustrates this principle of rapport in lower life.

In the animal world, wild creatures demonstrate a high ability of communication without the benefit of objective means, written language, or the spoken word.

And, of course, non-objective communication at the human level is a reality well-documented by ESP experience in every field. It may be as simple as a feeling of rapport between two close friends or as dramatic as the non-objective contact made between Mark and his wife on the Nevada desert. A universal principle of communication exists which gives rise to such phenomena. Furthermore, it is this same principle that makes verbal, visible, objective devices for communication possible.

Developing the faculty of metavision

What man needs now is a device for tapping and using his mental communication equipment. Instead of more video viewers, he needs a metaviewer. The Science of Higher Sense Perception provides such a device. The device, of course, involves no hardware. It is the technique for higher-sense reception through mind-training found in this chapter.

It is the technique I gave Dwight after he asked, "How do I become sensitive enough to get an HSP message in the first place?"

"Sensitivity," I explained to Dwight, "can be cultivated by developing your powers to visualize—to see with the mind instead of the eye. The physical eye can see only a surface world. The mind's eye can see causes, trends, underlying motivation, and inner factors.

The mind's eye can see beyond ordinary sight. Let's call this vision *insight, perception,* or better still, *metavision*—because it is a sight that is *meta* or *"higher than, beyond, and more comprehensive than physical vision."*

Dwight was willing to give sensitivity training a try. And, because he felt he had little skill at visualizing, I started him with an elementary technique. It is designed to condition the mind to watching, waiting, and looking for clairvoyant impressions. The person who is persistent in its practice may find himself highly successful in demonstrating expanded powers of self-guidance, self-direction, and insight.

First, train the mind to communicate with you in terms of pictures and mental images—train it to visualize. How? Make a METAVIEWER. Obtain a piece of black velvet cloth or black suede paper about 20 x 20 inches. Mount it in a frame so it will be sturdy enough to prop in front of you. Stand it on a chair or a low table that is level with your gaze and approximately four feet away. Sit in your special training chair for the session.

Second, assume the role of a META-SEER. Enter the session with the attitude that your mind's eye can see beyond and above the boundaries of physical vision. Affirm that you have the faculty to perceive in image-form hidden knowledge that can direct you toward right action, personal protection, guidance, and safety for loved ones.

Third, use the square of black velvet—your metaviewer—as the object of concentration as you work for sensitivity to mind's-eye perception. As metavision messages are usually in the form of communications between two people who are en rapport, make a friend or loved one the object of your concentration. Begin by gazing at the square of black velvet (for details, see the HSP Sensitivity Technique at the close of the chapter) and visualize your friend's face. Keep your attention on that image as you repeat the words, "Oneness, oneness—no space, no time separates us; we are one in mind."

Fourth, hold your gaze steadily on the metaviewer, or, if it is more comfortable, gradually let your eyes close. However, keep alert. Continue repeating the words above. As you quietly concentrate, become a beholder and a listener. You are an impersonal spectator, a meta-seer, seeing above and beyond the confines of the physical eye.

What are you watching and listening for? For the expanded knowledge and wisdom that can result from superior communication with your friend—knowledge that may manifest as an image on the metaviewer or a picture in your mind's eye.

Fifth, live expecting superior guidance and perception to come to you when you need it. Train yourself to be alert to clairvoyant reception. And, assure yourself that nothing but right-urges will come to you by using the following psi-programming pointer along with your sensitivity training for metavision.

Remember, Dwight had wondered, "How do I recognize an urge that can be trusted?"

You can trust impressions if you are sure they are the product of *higher* sense perception. And, you *can* be sure if you command the subconscious to screen out any urges that are not for your greater good.

Give this programmer as a command to your subconscious mind. Say it over three times slowly and forcefully. Repeat it often as you work with the techniques of metavision. As you condition the subconscious with this command, it will screen out impressions that are false, capricious, and meaningless, leaving only those which can be trusted.

Ψ   Psi-Programming Pointer
I AM A META-SEER VIEWING LIFE FROM AN EXPANDED LEVEL THAT MAKES MY SEEING CLEAR AND TRUE. I BEHOLD NOTHING FALSE FOR MY VISION IS THE PRODUCT OF *HIGHER* SENSE PERCEPTION.

A case of HSP guidance between friends

Sometime later, Dwight dropped into my office. I could tell from his inner excitement that he had something special to share.

He took from his pocket a newspaper clipping and, without

saying a word, handed it to me. It was the account of a hunter whose car had gone out of control. I read the article and handed it back.

"He's a friend of mine," Dwight explained. "Al Duggan and I have known each other for years, and I've gone hunting with him I don't know how many times!"

"I was with him on this trip, too," Dwight said, nodding toward the clipping, "except Duggan took his own car because he had to get back a day earlier than me. We left the city about 7:00 one morning and planned to meet at Schneider's Fork at noon. I hadn't filled my tank, so after I was on the road a half hour or so, I stopped for gas at Cedardale. Duggan honked and waved as he went past the station. When I pulled into Pine Ridge, I saw Duggan in the right lane behind some slow traffic. This time I passed him and we waved again."

Dwight's face grew serious as he continued. "I drove along for about an hour then, keeping my speed down and expecting to see Duggan's car behind me at any moment. As the miles rolled on, I got uneasy. The thought that something may have happened started gnawing at me. In my mind's eye I could see a car lying on its side."

"And, then," I prodded.

"I tried to put the thought out of my mind, but I remembered what you said in class about the woman who put the lamp in the window—HSP can't do you any good unless you *act* upon it. So, I turned my car around and went back. I didn't know exactly what I was looking for, but I drove slowly and watched each edge of the road. At a slight curve I saw some black tire marks that veered off to the shoulder. The curve was banked and hid the steep slope below it. I parked and walked to the brink. Below on its side was Duggan's car!"

I listened while Dwight took a deep breath and went on.

"I found Duggan unconscious and bleeding badly from a gash in his arm. I stopped the bleeding with a tourniquet and got help. They found that his brakes were defective. The thing is," Dwight declared, "that if I had driven clear to Schneider's Fork to meet Duggan at noon, he could have bled to death in the meantime, for his car was completely hidden from the road. Chances are that no one else would have discovered him."

I nodded, "HSP works, doesn't it!"

"You know," Dwight admitted, "until this happened, I really had no luck with the technique. However, Duggan was one of the friends whose face I used for concentration with the metaviewer. Nothing happened at the time, but this proves to me that rapport can be established and that it comes through as guidance and help when you need it."

"And when you *act* on it," I added.

Dwight's hunch was not spectacular. The results, however, were. The message came to him simply as a sense of uneasiness. Then, in his mind's eye he saw the accident. He scarcely knew whether the impression was his imagination or a real HSP urge, despite the fact that he had programmed a screening command into the subconscious.

In any event, Dwight felt it would do no harm to check out that hunch. How grateful he was that he did!

Why impressions come via various media

As you work with this book and develop your sensitivity to higher sense perception, you may find that one technique works better for you than another. HSP reception differs from one individual to another. As scores of case histories attest, one person may simply sense self-guidance as a feeling of uneasiness (premonition). Another may receive impressions visually (metavision). Still another may receive guidance as audible directions (metaudition).

Precognition, metavision, metaudition, and the like are simply the various media by which HSP reception may manifest, just as radio, telegraph, and television are electronic media. The center for all these different types of HSP reception is the *Tele-Data Receiver,* which picks up the signals and messages, no matter which of the various media is being used.

So it is with your higher sensory equipment: you have the ability through the higher use of mental laws to pick up HSP signals. These mental impulses may take various forms or manifest through various media. With the same essential equipment, you may receive clairvoyant hunches as Dwight did, premonitions, or telepathic messages.

Here are the media by which HSP impressions most frequently manifest, as explained in the Science of Higher Sense Perception:

Telepathy—is communication on an inner or non-verbal level. It corresponds to the spoken word on the outer, verbal level. Telepathy is non-objective communication; the spoken word is objective communication. Both are expressions of a basic thought-transmittal faculty—telepathy is its non-verbal form and speech is its verbal form.

Clairvoyance (metavision)—is a mental awareness that manifests as sight. It is vision that is independent of the physical eye. The word, traced back to Latin, comes from *clarus* and *videre* meaning *"to see clearly."* Clairvoyance is perception that extends beyond the range of physical vision. Therefore, in this book it is termed *metavision*—higher vision.

Clairaudience (metaudition)—is an interior cognition that manifests as sound or the spoken word. It is independent of the physical auditory nerve. *Audience,* the *"act or state of hearing,"* comes from the Latin word *audire* meaning *"to hear."* With *clarus,* it becomes *"clear hearing."* In this study, you will find the faculty of "clear hearing" referred to as *metaudition*—higher hearing—a medium through which expanded perception may register.

Precognition—is a sensing which is independent of time. It is predicting the future and the shape of things to come as prophesied by present trends. It is foreseeing such trends and their consequences prior to their manifestation in the time-space world. When precognition carries a sense of forewarning or foreboding, it is termed premonition.

Retrocognition—is, likewise, a knowing which is independent of time. It is the sensing of experiences and causes that have already taken place. Retrocognition deals with former situations from the historical past, but it is a *present viewing* of that past. It is like seeing a television show which was filmed yesterday but is viewed today.

Telekinesis—is an ability to influence and control objects at a distance from the physical self without the use of physical means. *Kinesis* is a Greek word meaning *"to move or motion,"* and *tele* means *"far off; at a distance."*

Actually, the mind functions in a telekinetic role in normal, daily performance. The mind moves the body by remote control whenever it gets you up in the morning, sits you down to eat, or walks you to work. But, because of the closeness of your mental self to the body, you have the feeling that the body is moving itself by physical means alone.

Still other types of phenomena

There are a number of other types of phenomena or other media through which impressions may manifest. One is the **awareness of impending death** which may be considered to be a type of precognition.

Another is the appearance of **stigmata**. Temporary stigmata—bodily marks, brands, or wounds—sometimes manifest as a result of religious ecstasy. Deep empathy and emotionalism have much to do with such phenomena. For example, a person vicariously reliving the Crucifixion may so vividly experience a reenactment of the event that wounds resembling nail holes appear on the hands. This phenomenon results form the interaction of such factors as retrocognition and telekinesis.

Another phenomenon is **automatism or automatic writing**. This faculty sometimes manifests as an invisible force which moves a person's hand across the page as he writes uncontrollably. It sometimes manifests as slatewriting where chalk seemingly moves by itself on the surface of a slate hidden from view in a shallow box. This phenomenon results from the action of telekinetic power motivated by psychical impressions.

A case of expanded sense of smell

There is still another type of higher sense perception which, to coin a phrase, is referred to below as metaolfaction. Keep in mind the definition of *meta* as *"higher or beyond; transcending,"* while *olfaction* is *"the sense of smell; the process of smelling." Metaolfaction,* thus, is higher sensory perception that manifests as an impression of smell.

This case illustrates the phenomenon of metaolfaction. Mary B. enrolled in a course on meditation techniques. During the series of lectures, the leader told his class how to concentrate upon an object to keep the mind from wandering. To sustain concentration on one idea for five minutes, the class members were to take something like a seed. "Hold it in your hand," he advised, "and see it send down a root and sprout a tiny leaf. Visualize it spreading out into a plant. Imagine the blossoms unfolding. As they fade, see the seed pods form and ripen. Then, visualize the new seed being sown and becoming the next harvest—again and again, until the world is covered."

Returning from the class, Mary decided to practice her newly learned concentration technique. She sat quietly in her living room and selected a rose for the object of her visualization. She pictured herself holding a dormant bareroot rose. She saw it rooting and sending out its tender green leaves. She imagined it growing and spreading out upon a trellis. Then, rose buds swelled on the bush and broke out into a riot of blossoms covering the trellis from bottom to top.

Mary completed her meditation and went to the kitchen to prepare dinner for her husband. Returning to the living room a few minutes later, she found the room heavy with the scent of roses. It was not the season out-of-doors for roses, and there were no cut flowers in the room. The fragrance was so pronounced, however, that she found it overpowering. She had to open the window to air the room.

If it seems strange that mental roses could throw off such a scent, it is well to remember how powerful an idea can be. If a rose-consciousness can exist, a thorn-consciousness can also exist, and you can create *either* depending on the direction you give your thoughts.

To a great extent, you will generally hear what your consciousness permits you to hear and generally see what your consciousness permits you to see. To see a richer world, you must entertain thoughts that permit you to enjoy a *wealth of feeling*.

Using your different sensory receptors

The media through which HSP impressions register are probably connected with the individuality of the perceiver himself. Certainly, when it comes to broadcast reception, one person may have an inclination to listen to radio and another may prefer watching television. The radio listener will *hear;* the TV viewer will *see*.

So, too, when it comes to higher sensory reception, one person may be susceptible to impressions that manifest as audible warnings while another is more sensitive to guidance in visual form. Doubtlessly, the person who is skillful at visualization is more likely to receive metavision impressions than the individual who has little visualizing skill.

Hence, factors in the psychic and mental constitution of the individual may make one perceiver clairvoyant, another clairaudient, and still another telepathic.

However, the woman who concentrated on roses and had the metaolfactory experience *also* frequently experienced instances of clairvoyant guidance and telepathy. She is not unique, so the conclusion must be that HSP is not necessarily limited to one medium of manifestation. Life has created five different sensory receptors for the purpose of a wide range of awareness at the physical level. The range must be even greater at the expanded level of higher sense perception. *Any and all* HSP powers can be cultivated by you to a significant degree.

Metavision is no impossible dream

The essential questions are: how do you cultivate HSP powers? How do you become sensitive to higher sensory media? More specifically, because this chapter deals with metavision, how do you develop higher seeing?

The answer is that you must work at it and work systematically and scientifically. Manifestation of the higher use of the principles of Mind cannot be left to chance happening.

If television had been left to the chance happening of the laws of electronics, how long would the world have waited for the development of the video tube?

Or, if science had relegated the concept of television to the junk heap as an impossible dream, how likely would its invention have been?

The development of higher sensory powers is no impossible dream. Do not leave it to chance happening. Cultivate it systematically. It requires expanding your concepts, your expectations, your vision and faith. It requires a grasp of new ways to put known laws to work at higher levels.

The possibility of metavision is no more a violation of mental law than television is a violation of the law of electronics. When you sit in your living room a hundred miles—perhaps three thousand miles—from Washington and watch the President of the United States give a speech from the White House, your eye catching every movement of his lips and expression of his face, is your experience a violation of the principle of vision?

Of course, the answer is NO! Yet, 19th century man would have thought it insane to believe that one day such an event would be shared by millions of people at the same moment. However, man's expanding knowledge of the law of electronics has made television a common reality for all. Similarly, one day an expanding knowledge of the laws of Mind can make metavision a common experience.

Every day and every decade reveal new wonders that emerge as man delves more deeply into the nature of the universe and its laws.

There was a time when man believed that ships had to be made of wood, for wood floated while iron sank. This, it seemed, was a law. Then, it was discovered that iron would float if the weight of the water displaced was greater than the weight of the displacing object. This refinement was not a violation of law but simply a higher use of a known law. The law of physics did not change to permit iron to float, but man's *application* of the law changed.

There was a time, and not so long ago, when it was believed that heavier-than-air machines could not possibly fly. Today, millions of miles of air travel attest to the fact that man *can* fly! When a jet pilot takes off from Los Angeles and an hour or two later finds himself in New York, he has no thought that he has done something mysterious or abnormal. But, he *has* used a law about which man knew little a century ago—the law of aerodynamics.

What you will be doing in the Science of Higher Sense Perception is to learn new applications of known powers—powers that may seem at first like impossible dreams, as impossible as the iron ship which floats. What you will be doing is putting known laws to extended uses of which traditional uses are but a small part.

Factors involved in clairvoyant transmission

A few paragraphs from now you will actually be putting mental laws to an extended use. You will actually undertake training with your metaviewer. A striking similarity exists between metavision and television, and seeing it will help you grasp what you are doing.

Think of metavision as the non-objective, mental counterpart of television. Sending and receiving concepts are involved in both, and transmission must be synchronized.

Metavision transmission is dependent upon a sender and receiver (perceiver). The message sent must be synchronized. That is, the message projected by a sender will not register unless (or until) the perceiver is receptive (for there is such a thing as delayed reception).

Television transmission, of course, is likewise dependent upon sending and receiving an image and upon synchronization. In projecting a television image from one place to another, the light intensity of a scene is converted into electrical signals. This is accomplished by a scanner connected with the iconoscope at the sending-end which picks up the image line-by-line and transmits it across the miles. At the receiving-end, the kinescope scanner, *synchronized* with the first scanner, reassembles the impulses into the original image.

A dictionary defines *synchronicity* as *"happening, existing, or arising at or about the same time."* This synchronicity must exist between the sender and perceiver of a metavisional image. Some way, they must be attuned or en rapport. Often they are husband and wife as was the case with Mark, or daughter and father as was the case with Carolyn in Chapter Two. Or, they may be friends as was true of Dwight and Duggan.

Almost always the perceiver is in a receptive, quiescent state—in idle thought, quiet activity, meditation, or sleep. Transmittal of the sender's message must synchronize with the perceiver's receptive state, if the image is to be received.

Mark's wife was sleeping and receptive when his desperate feeling, "I must get home," was transmitted.

Carolyn was quiet and receptive at the kitchen window when the accident befell her father. Her brother's first thought was to get his father home, and she perceived it. She *saw* what was wrong.

Dwight was quietly driving along a mountain road when Duggan's plight was transmitted to him.

There are times, of course, when it appears that no sender is involved in clairvoyant experiences. However, who can say what unspoken thoughts flash through the minds of those present at dramatic scenes or what intensity of feeling even a spectator may experience? Clairvoyant transmission is seldom a deliberate, fully conscious act.

Psychological preparation for metaviewing

Your success in developing clairvoyant powers will depend largely on attitude—your own and others. If you are skeptical and doubt your ability to use HSP powers, you are psychologically prepared to fail. If others around you are uninformed regarding psi-power and deny the world beyond their five senses, they create psychological blocks that hamper you also.

Skepticism is a definite hindrance to success in any area. If you belittle your ability, your talents, and your self-confidence, then you curtail your effectiveness no matter what field you are in.

Skepticism acts as a special block to higher sensory skills. You must prepare yourself psychologically for success with faith and a willingness to try the techniques in this book. You must have a feeling that HSP powers are logical, normal, and your rightful possession.

Equally disastrous as your own skepticism is the criticism of others. When someone challenges your convictions and asks you to prove their validity, negative vibrations result. Avoid others who cannot look behind the testimony of the five senses and realize that an extended world exists of which the known world is but a small part. On the other hand, *do* cultivate those who can believe that there are unexplored mental realms to tap and higher uses of known laws to discover.

To help you condition yourself to expect results in demonstrating psi-power and prepare yourself psychologically, use the following psi-programming pointer. It will program your subconscious mind with a success attitude which neutralizes criticism, doubt, and skepticism.

Ψ   Psi-Programming Pointer
HE WHO DENIES EXTENDED SENSORY POWERS IS
DENYING THE GREATER PART OF HIS POTENTIAL. AS
FOR ME, I NOW PREPARE TO TAP THAT POTENTIAL WITH
AN ATTITUDE OF DISCOVERY, EXPECTANCY, AND
FAITH.

STEPS IN DEVELOPING METAVISION

Metavisional pathways of communication

To develop your sensitivity to superior guidance and perception when you need it, practice beforehand the ability to visualize. By encouraging your mind to see in *image-form* those with whom you are en rapport (friends and loved ones), you can establish silent pathways of communication over which guidance can come.

First: As the principle of metavision requires a sender and receiver who are attuned, choose for each of your experiments in metavision someone to whom you are close. Prepare yourself comfortably for contemplation with the metaviewer explained in detail earlier in this chapter. If your powers of visualization are good, picture your friend's face as you gaze into the square of black velvet. If you are not skillful with mental imagery, start by looking at a snapshot of your friend. Then, transfer your gaze from the snapshot to the velvet and retain his image in your mind's eye.

Second: With your gaze fixed on the square, think of yourself as a meta-seer. Think of yourself as one who can see beyond this physical dimension. Affirm that you have the faculty of higher sight. As you concentrate on the image of your friend's face, maintain an attitude of watchful waiting. You are waiting for superior knowledge—for expanded awareness or wisdom your friend may wish to share with you.

Third: There is no force, no strain involved. You do not insist on communicating. You are establishing a metavisional pathway *now* which may carry a message to you at a *later time* when communication is important. Do not let the concentration be taxing.

Choose one friend and use his face as an object of concentration for several days. Start with ten-minute sessions twice a day and build up to a half hour.

Fourth: Realize that your higher self speaks in its own language which, for the most part, is the language of symbolism. When images appear on your metaviewer, they are likely to be similar to the symbolic presentations of a dream state. How do you interpret them? This depends, for symbols are strictly personal to you. Symbols are the voice of your own subconscious mind. It will be helpful to become familiar with certain basic ones as discussed in Chapter Eight—fire, water, the vine, certain animals, etc.—yet their significance will depend on your own personality. Affirm that you will *know* the meaning of the symbolic images and messages that come to you.

Fifth: Develop metavisional rapport with those who are important to your happiness and well-being by practicing the detailed method given in HSP Sensitivity Training Technique No. 3. Read the technique a time or two until you can follow it and *feel* it as an experience in consciousness.

HSP-SENSITIVITY TRAINING TECHNIQUE NO. 3

PRACTICING THE ART OF METAVISION

You settle yourself now in your chair reserved for psi-training, relax, and breathe deeply several times. To induce a contemplative mood, you remember the two previous trips-in-consciousness you had in this same chair.

During these trips, the DOOR OF LIFE opened unto you and gave you a glimpse of the oneness of things. You recapture the oneness you felt as your eyes followed the solitary cloud that blended with the vastness of the sky. You feel that your mind, like the cloud, is blending with the vastness of Universal Mind. You feel that you are one with something bigger than yourself. Your vision expands! Your awareness increases! You are attuned to like minds!

You sustain this expanded feeling of oneness and attunement as you fix your gaze upon the deep, velvety square of your meta viewer. In your mind's eye, you see the face of your friend.

You trace every detail of his features clearly, visualizing the hair style, the contour of the forehead and cheek, the color of eyes, shape of the nose, roundness of the lip, and tilt of the chin. You mentally picture each highlight and each shadow.

You keep your mind blank and free from all directed thoughts. You interiorize your level of attention. Your gaze is steady and you concentrate upon the picture before your mind's eye. If your concentration strays, bring it back, silently repeating over and over, *"Oneness . . . Oneness . . . Oneness."*

You now wipe out the time and space boundaries of the physical level and establish greater rapport with your friend by affirming, *"No space, no time, separates us; we are one in Mind."*

With your eyes still on the black square, or with eyes closed, feel that the blackness grows in depth until it becomes a window opening out into the infinite. You are a meta-seer, a beholder, an expectant spectator, gazing through that window. You wait patiently. You are not *trying* for anything; you are *letting.* You are letting a higher vision penetrate a level of expanded awareness.

Now, images in your mind's eye may appear in the window of your metaviewer. They may be fleeting scenes or symbolic presentations. To you, they are meaningful. They are significant. They increase your wisdom and understanding.

Now, you relax your gaze and your concentration. You let the vision of your friend's face fade in a feeling of warmth and high regard for him. You affirm that a metavisional pathway of rapport exists between you that will serve as a means of constructive communication when needed—a pathway of mutual blessing, guidance, and understanding.

Hold this thought in silence for a moment and then end your training session by decreeing:

And so it is!

SUMMARY CAPSULES

YOUR HIGHER SENSE OF METAVISION

Residing in the interior of your Self right now is the higher sense of metavision. It is the operation of the principle of sight functioning above the physical level. It is a part of your consciousness-equipment and is waiting to be tapped by you. *No eye*

one—and precognition and retrocognition become experiences natural to that larger view.

Your four basic relationships with life

Although they are natural, precognition and retrocognition seem to be outside the realm of normal experience. Why? . . . because normal experience is dominated by the physical. You give most of your time and attention to the body bobbing up and down in the canoe on the River of Life.

The physical self, of course, is part of *what* and *who* you are. However, your relationship with the physical is only one of four relationships you have with life. To become preoccupied with this relationship is to restrict yourself to *objective perceptions* arising from the five physical senses alone. You should be cognizant of all four relationships you have with life:

First, there is your relationship with your body. You are not your body, although the tie is intimate. Your body is an instrument for your use. In the very fact that you can say, "I have a body," lies the inescapable conclusion that there is something superior to the body which says, "I."

Second, there is your relationship to the external world around you, to other people, things, objective conditions, to your work, and to the environmental factors in your daily life.

Third, there is your relationship to your Self—not to your objective body, but to the mental *being of eternity* you really are. This is the internal world of thought, feeling, ideas, patterns, attitudes, and consciousness.

Fourth, is your relationship to that creative power from which your real Self springs. This is your intimate tie with the Creative Mind that is the parent cause of you.

Give attention to the paramount relationship

Evaluating the *interest* you give these four relationships, how would you rate your attention from a percentage standpoint? Thinking in terms of 100 per cent for all four, what amount of time do you give to the *first*—to maintaining your body? In your consideration, take into account feeding your body three or more times daily, washing it, assuaging its thirst. Take into account exercising it, entertaining it, clothing it, keeping it warm, putting it to bed, and catering to its comfort. Would the time spent on physical concerns amount to 60 or 70 per cent of your attention?

What percentage of time would you allot to your *second* relationship—to your objective world—relationships with friends, family, your work, the theater, television, newspapers, and books? Would the time spent on these concerns amount to 25 or 30 per cent of your attention?

If so, this would leave a possible 5 per cent for the *third* and *fourth* relationships—to your real Self and to the Creative Mind from which you spring.

Many are quick to dismiss the significance of HSP or higher sense perception. Isn't it because they give such a small percentage of their concern to their relationship with these last two areas?

What basis does a critic have for affirming that higher dimensions of mind do not exist when he is mired so deeply in the material world that he can see no other. To the person who has developed no relationship with the higher-sense Self and knows nothing of its power, it should be said "If you haven't tried it, don't knock it."

How you can break the time-sense barrier

Why has man generally been restricted to normal experiences, missing out on the vast realm of higher-than-normal powers potential to him?

Basically, it is because man's life is nurtured in objective sense perceptions. The earth is his mother, and he is tied to her apron strings in time-sense ways. He needs to gain a new perspective that will enable him to break the time-sense barrier.

Second, things as they appear to be (objective things) have an hypnotic hold over man's mind and the ideas he entertains. It is difficult to entertain a new idea when hypnotized by a traditional concept. For example, a short time ago, man believed the earth was flat and was the center of the universe. It appeared to be that way!

He believed that ships had to be made of wood, for wood floated while iron sank. It appeared to be that way!

Progress comes when man breaks free of old suggestions and old appearances. Advancement awaits his refusal to accept things as they appear to be. Man will be limited to the confines of his idea-world until he challenges the truth of appearances around him. Like an animal tethered to a stake, he is free to move only within the limits of his idea-world.

Taking your cue from this, you must build a larger idea-world. You must discard the old time-concept that defines today as a thin slice of eternity wedged between yesterday and tomorrow. You must break free of the suggestion that your powers are limited to what they appear to be at the present. Then, you must develop an expansive concept of time realizing that, from a higher dimension of consciousness, the past, present and future may be viewed as one.

Thus, you will find yourself acquiring new insight into things in your everyday world. Greater foresight and self-guidance will manifest for you. Things which seem to be problems at the moment, things which trouble you and give you concern, will suddenly be clear. You will see both the *cause* and the *solution,* for you will have the BIG VIEW (like the self on the rim of the canyon.)

To build the habit of rising in your imagination to a more lofty view of your world—to help you become time-free rather than time-bound—use the following Psi-Programming Pointer.

Ψ   Psi-Programming Pointer
MENTALLY I CLIMB UNTIL THE PAST, PRESENT, AND FUTURE BLEND INTO THE "BIG VIEW" AND A NEW SENSE OF INSIGHT BECOMES MINE.

What supernormal and supernatural mean

There is a higher world, a realm of principle, that is the cause of the world you see. The visible world is not an illusion, but it is an effect of that which is higher. The world of *invisible* principle that is back of the *visible* contains infinite possibilities. It has no limitations, no confines. It is the great unfenced potential.

Supernormal perception is the direct use of the principles of this higher invisible world. This does not imply something supernatural, however. Do not confuse the word *supernormal* with the word *supernatural*. *Supernormal* means *"exceeding the normal or average; being beyond usual human powers; paranormal."* The word *supernatural*, although close in definition, suggests something that violates nature—something unnatural.

Therefore, in the Science of Higher Sense Perception, a distinction is made between these two words. HSP phenomena may be defined as being supernormal or paranormal, but they are not unnatural. They are not a violation of natural law. Rather, they are proof of a higher extension of natural law. All phenomena can be explained when the higher law by which they manifest is understood.

There is an infinite range of qualities and values *beyond* the *normal sensory range* of perception. These qualities may appear *super-normal* while being perfectly *natural* to the above-normal dimension on which they manifest.

Limitations of four-dimensional perception

The plane on which precognition and retrocognition take place *appears to be above normal* for man is so accustomed to experiences that occur within the four dimensions he has known.

He measures and locates most things in four-dimensional terms. A straight line represents the first dimension—LENGTH. Using it to locate a meeting spot, one friend may say to another, "I'll meet you on Main Street."

However, Main Street is long, and to make the meeting place more specific, the friend may answer, "Make that at the intersection of Main and Lincoln." Two streets or two lines intersecting represent two dimensions—LENGTH and WIDTH.

Now, if a highrise happens to be on the corner specified for the meeting, a third dimension comes into consideration—HEIGHT. On what floor of the building will the friends meet?

Finally, they may still miss each other unless a time for the appointment is set. TIME is the fourth familiar dimension.

It is this fourth dimension that plays tricks on man. It seems to start for him at birth and end at death. A day seems to start with dawn and end with dusk. This is only because man has a limited concept of time. It would be more accurate to say that man lives in an *unlimited* time-dimension but that he has evolved only a *limited perception* of it.

As that perception grows for a person, he becomes aware of new, expansive concepts of time. He becomes the real Self on the mesa rim, and he gets a glimpse of some of the things that are natural to that above-normal level. Belonging to that expanded dimension are such faculties as intuition, precognition, and retro-cognition. From the rim, he can see *what the future course of his canoe will be* and *where it came from in the past.*

Potentialities of the fifth dimension

To gain the big view and the expanded insight it brings, you must train yourself to see beyond ordinary height, depth, breadth, and time concepts.

For example, let us say that ordinarily you are like an observer in a three-dimensional room, representing SPACE (height, length, and width). That room is a large hall with a window at either end. A bird enters the hall through one of the windows. As it comes in through the opening, you say that it is born.

As it passes through the room, you observe it. It appears to exist, to belong.

As it vanishes out the window at the far end, its existence seems to end. You call its disappearance death or extinction.

The passing of the bird through the room—marked by its birth, existence, and death—symbolizes the ordinary concept of TIME. Time is that which passes; most of it lies in the past or in the future.

How does this traditional concept differ from an expanded HSP concept of time?

Again, think of yourself as an observer in that same hall. Only this time, your view is expanded and you can see *beyond* the window through which the bird will enter the hall. As you observe him, he glides from tree to tree in the world outside the window.

Then, as before, the bird enters the open window and flies through the hall, leaving at the far end. Only this time, his disappearance is not death, for—with your expanded vision—you can still see him winging his way skyward.

The HSP concept of TIME extends beyond the walls of the hall, making yesterday and tomorrow a part of a present today. Thus, time does not lie in the past or future, but in the present. This view of time creates a new unlimited time-dimension, a *fifth dimension*. To see into that fifth dimension is to look out of the windows at both ends of the hall and see past, present, and future NOW.

With HSP training, the past and future can become timeless realms that may be perceived from where you stand in the present. Figuratively, you can enter an unlimited time-dimension that gives you the "big view" of things.

The possibility of probing the future carries with it superb potentialities of insight. This, Craig demonstrated. The possibility of tapping the past carries with it astonishing potentialities of knowledge. This, Wilma demonstrated.

How retrocognition solved a personal problem

Wilma J. came to me one night after class. She looked tired and dejected. It didn't take long to get the story.

"It's my son's new wife," Wilma said. "I do so want Jim and her to get off to a good start. I try to please her, but she is hostile towards me. If I just understood why!"

"Try to get that big view," I suggested, "the one I've been talking about in class. Just as it can help through foresight to make you aware of future trends, it can help through retrosight to make you aware of past motivation and causes."

I recommended that Wilma use a psi-programmer to open her mind to the knowledge that retrocognition could bring her. Adjustment between her and her daughter-in-law would be easier if she could find the hidden cause of the hostility. Empathy and forgiveness spring from retrocognitive perception. You can understand most any viewpoint and make allowance for it if you know the cause behind it.

The wry comment that "it's easy to have perfect 20-20 vision with hindsight" is all too true. *Without the ability* to look behind present scenes for past causes, a person's mental vision is far from perfect. *With the ability*, however, you can demonstrate 20-20 perception and avoid many heartaches, misunderstandings, and wrong conclusions.

Wilma took the psi-programming command I gave her and agreed to program it into her subconscious mind. This she did in periods of quiet contemplation each morning for a week. She had learned in class that spaced daily repetition firmly fixes a command in the subconscious. In the evening just as she retired, she practiced the more formal training given in the HSP Sensitivity techniques at the end of this chapter. Her command to the subconscious was a *request for understanding* through insight and retrocognition.

Then, an amazing thing happened. One afternoon Wilma took her dog for a walk in a nearby park. It was a lazy day, and when she came to an empty bench, she sat down. She idly watched her dog for a few minutes; her thoughts were on nothing in particular.

Suddenly, the park seemed to change to a garden someplace. She "saw" two women facing each other—one was quite young. As the scene became clear, Wilma recognized the young one. It was her new daughter-in-law.

The two women were arguing violently. Wilma heard only one phrase distinctly, but it echoed and re-echoed in her mind. "You're to blame," the young woman screamed. "You broke up my marriage with Michael. You're the typical bossy, selfish, possessive, domineering mother-in-law!"

The vision faded as quickly as it came, and Wilma sat stunned on the bench. For a few long, puzzled moments she searched for some meaning to it all.

She knew that her daughter-in-law had been married before. Could it be that her former husband was named Michael? If so, the meaning of Wilma's retrocognitive vision was clear. She had become the target for animosity created by a former mother-in-law.

Wilma called her dog and hurried home. She made some discreet telephone inquiries and found that "yes" her daughter-in-law had been married to a "Michael." Wilma understood now. She felt a surge of compassion toward her son's new wife, and she vowed never to become a bossy, interfering mother-in-law herself.

Retrocognitive insight need not manifest in a form as dramatic as that experienced by Wilma. Often such perception comes simply as a feeling, a knowingness, an awareness. Here is a psi-programming command that can help you develop this kind of retrocognitive awareness. Use it, as Wilma did, when you need guidance and understanding on personal problems.

Ψ   Psi-Programming Pointer

MY VISION IS NOW BIGGER THAN TIME. IT STRETCHES EASILY INTO THE PAST TO BRING ME A NEW DIMENSION OF UNDERSTANDING AND INSIGHT INTO THE CAUSE OF THINGS.

What makes retrocognition possible?

What made it possible for Wilma to witness what she did? In what psychic *form* do past events persist? What universal laws of higher sense perception are involved?

Raynor Johnson, in *The Imprisoned Splendour,* suggests that the past may exist as a persistent memory on the psychic plane. To illustrate his point, he tells of the retrocognitive experience of Edith Oliver.

The place was England; the date was October, 1916. Miss Oliver was driving a small car from Devizes to Swindom in Wiltshire near dusk. It was between 5:00 and 6:00 P.M. and a gentle rain was falling. She loved the rain, and her mood was quiet and meditative.

Soon she found she had left the main road and was passing along a strange avenue with huge, grey megaliths standing on either side. She assumed that she was approaching Avebury. She had never visited here before, but she recognized it from pictures she had seen in archeological books.

Now she was driving up a stone avenue. Arriving at the end of it, she climbed out and saw more huge megaliths standing and fallen in an irregular fashion, with cottages interspersed among them. A village fair seemed to be in progress although it was still drizzling. She saw flares and torches lighting the booths, various shows in progress, primitive swing-boats, and strolling groups of villagers. The rain became heavier, so Miss Oliver got back in her car and drove on.

Nine years later, Miss Oliver visited Avebury with a friend. She learned that Avebury had once had annual fairs, but she was astonished that they had not been held since 1850. The next year when again visiting the region as a member of a society studying the strange monument, she discovered to her amazement that the avenue of megaliths up which she believed she had come on her first visit had disappeared before the year 1800. It would seem that on that rainy evening in October, 1916, she had viewed a scene which took place over a century before.

Commenting on this, Raynor Johnson says, "This type of experience suggests a kind of persistent memory in the psychic ether associated with a place, to which in a certain receptive state of mind a sensitive person may tune-in."[1]

The retro-cinematography process

The "persistent memory in the psychic ether" of which Johnson speaks has been called the psychic record. Think of that record as being akin to the image made when a motion-picture is filmed.

The original action of a drama on a Hollywood sound stage, once performed, persists as a record upon the sensitized celluloid strip to which the action was exposed. Similarly, human dramas, once performed, persist as a record in the sensitized medium of Mind. Yes, universal Mind is something like a reel of movie film upon which the past has etched itself through a process of retro-cinematography. Hence, the *past* is *present* now as a memory record.

The possibility of *past events* existing as a form of *present record* is no more startling than what is being done experimentally with infrared light in the field of photography.

During the Cuban missile crises in 1962, newspapers across the nation carried a headline proclaiming: "CAMERA THAT CAN PHOTOGRAPH PAST EVENTS USED IN CUBA." The press reported that, "The airbourne infrared 'eye' (of the camera), operated electronically, can look down at night from an altitude of more than 40,000 feet to a place on earth, such as a Cuban missile site, and reflect images of people and equipment *not then present* but on the site earlier in the day."[2]

---

[1] Johnson, Raynor C. *The Imprisoned Splendor*. New York: Harper & Row, Publishers, Inc., 1953, p. 160.

[2] *The Denver Post*. Denver, Colorado, October 25, 1962.

Thus, in the field of photography, man has achieved that which seemed impossible before. Making higher use of known laws of light, he finds he can photograph past events. By the same token, by the higher use of known laws of mind, man can perceive past events. The infrared camera eye can see events which took place earlier in the day. With the mental eye of expanded vision, man can perceive events which took place *"earlier in the day"* of time.

Edith Oliver perceived events in the psychic record that took place at Avebury much, much "earlier in the day"—to be exact, 100 years earlier. Wilma J. perceived events that had taken place only a year or so earlier. Is there any limit to how far you can roll back the film of time?

To answer this, think again of the process of past events impressing themselves as lasting records on a motion-picture type medium of Mind—the process of retro-cinematography. Think of yourself as the retro-viewer. Is there any reason you could not re-run the moving memory-picture back to any place in history?

Establishing a timeless relationship to life

Your relationship with the universe is not a *time relationship.* It is a *timeless one;* it exists in the NOW. There *has never been* more of life than there is now. There *will never be* more of life than there is now. Learn to utilize life now to the fullest of your potentialities!

There is a timeless reality back of all time. There is a changeless reality back of all change. The Science of Higher Sense Perception beckons you to expand your awareness of this timeless and changeless source of power. However, your sense perception is time-oriented. You are, by this very fact, inclined to think in terms of events as being at a distance from you time-wise. It is typical to feel that success is evading you just beyond your grasp. It is normal to feel that fulfillment is still around the corner. But such an attitude serves only to postpone success and fulfillment.

Events, experiences, and conditions are not located in time but in consciousness. You live in consciousness. Consciousness is like a revolving sphere rolling along the horizontal track of time. Experience takes place within that sphere rather than in time. As Henri Bergson says in *Creative Evolution,* "My mental state, as it advances on the road of time, is continually swelling with the duration which it accumulates."[3] This *duration which accumulates* is consciousness.

A dictionary defines *consciousness* as *"awareness; the state of being characterized by sensation, emotion, volition, and thought: MIND; the totality of conscious states."* In HSP, consciousness means this sum total of the individual's awareness into which is incorporated his attitudes, values, subjective memories, opinions, understandings, and—hopefully—expanded concepts of his real Self.

As Bergson implies, consciousness is cumulative. It builds with duration as it moves along in time. However, consciousness itself is essentially timeless. It is the sphere within which you live—within which your life revolves—as that sphere rolls along the time-track.

You live in consciousness. Hence, that which belongs to your consciousness is never lost or left behind—unless, of course, you release it. Positive qualities that belong to consciousness need never disappear.

Learning to live in the present

Unfortunately, many people *do* feel that what belongs to them has been lost and left behind. How common it is for an individual to feel that an opportunity of which he did not take advantage is irretrievably lost! How often a person pines for some friend who is gone or a way-of-life that is over!

However, when you learn to live in *consciousness* instead of in time, you will find that the potentialities of life—of *all* life—are present now. Happiness and friends need not belong to a past that is dead and gone! Success need not belong to an evasive future which never comes!

Good friends, companionship, and success can belong to you as much today as ever. They belong to the consciousness you are. Once you have them in consciousness, they cannot be lost, left behind, or forsaken.

---

[3]Bergson, Henri, *Creative Evolution.* New York: Holt, Rinehart and Winston, Inc , 1944, p. 4.

The secret of personal power lies in building a consciousness equal to the values you wish to experience. In a companion book, *The Science of Mental Cybernetics*, techniques for building such a consciousness are given in detial.

A case study in time mastery

Nora was saying to me, "But my friends are all gone. I could name dozens of people I once knew who have passed on. I'll never see them again. There was a lawyer whose judgment I could always rely on and so many other worth-while friends who are gone now!"

As we talked, I was aware that Nora W. had a problem that troubles many people—a sense of loss. Time had stolen her friends. Similar is the sense of loss people feel when success disappears into the past. Time has robbed them. Time is also the culprit that stands between many and their future dreams. They long with desperation for a day that will bring better things.

Nora, and all who feel a sense of loss, need to develop the mental ability to *master* time instead of serving as a *victim* of its passage. I talked with her about this. "Where do you think the love and friendships you had existed?" I asked her. "Did they exist in *time* or in *consciousness?*"

Nora looked puzzled, so I continued. "Granted, certain people you once knew as names, personalities, and companions, are no longer physically here. But you had them as friends because of a quality of consciousness. Your consciousness attracted the companionship you knew, and what belongs to your consciousness cannot be lost."

"I wish I could believe that," Nora sighed.

"Look at it this way," I said. "Where is the consciousness that brought you your friends of yesterday? Did you leave it behind in some time-track year such as 1960 or 1970? Did you lose it back in Chicago or San Diego? Were your friendships something that could only happen once? Wasn't it your consciousness that created them? Wasn't it a state of consciousness that lived and loved? Of course, it was! And it is the same consciousness that can re-create the companionship you want now!

"The main thing is not to let time trick you into thinking that the past holds all of your good. You can master time—you can demonstrate dominion over it—by affirming that your good exists in the eternal NOW. It is resident in the consciousness in which you presently live."

I would like to report that Nora left my desk, went out immediately, and made new friends. It didn't work quite that fast, but she did realize now that friendship and companions belonged to her because her consciousness attracted them. She stopped bemoaning her lost loves of the past and grew more optimistic about the present. It was not long thereafter that she formed some outstanding new friendships.

You can do what Nora did. She realized that the past had not robbed her of anything. All of the values she had ever had were present with her in the NOW. Without delay, she began to use those values to enrich her life.

STEPS IN THE MASTERY OF TIME

First, to demonstrate dominion over the past, don't leave your future behind you in your attempt to retrieve some happy experience. Hold on to a fond recollection as memory-wealth, but don't long for it as though it can never be manifested again. Your consciousness called forth the experiences of yesterday— experiences that belonged to you. *This* it will continue to do, for life must manifest that for which your inner mental pattern calls.

Second, the future of your life resides in the idea-germ of today. Nothing exists tomorrow that does not stir unborn in consciousness now. Conceive today the self-image you wish to demonstrate. Nurture the idea. Incorporate it into your consciousness, and it will become the experience of your future.

Third, to free your mind from the pressure of time, learn to think of each moment as part of a present eternity You are living in a *here and now* which is eternally present. True, time is a track, but you live in a sphere which revolves along that track. And, although time passes, there is a timelessness within that sphere-of-consciousness. Here you will find the *present eternity* you need to achieve all your dreams, your ambitions, and your heart's desire.

Fourth, don't let your mind dwell on old experience for this may bar a new future. If you cease to be creative, the great sleep begins. If you cease to grow, the mind turns in upon itself and consciousness plays a memory record of monotony. Static tunes of consciousness must inevitably repeat so long as the individual lives at the same level of experience.

Fifth, use the following HSP Sensitivity Training Technique to gain a feeling of release from the demands of time. In your mind's eye, become that lofty observer on the mesa rim who, in one sweep, beholds the past, present, and future as a unit in a larger dimension.

HSP-SENSITIVITY TRAINING TECHNIQUE NO. 4

YOU, BEHOLDER OF THE BIG VIEW

Be seated in your chair, relax, breathe deeply and free your mind from the cares of the moment. In your imagination, picture yourself standing on a path at the foot of an immense mountain. You cannot see very far back down the trail from whence you came for it turns and twists. Your view ahead is blocked by the steep valley walls stretching upward. Although your view at this point is limited, what you see invites you forward.

You begin to ascend the mountain. There is no sense of strain. You move forward easily, confidently, and light of step. As the climb becomes steeper, you begin to see beyond the limiting confines of the lower trail. As you continue, you reach a level where you can now see the path behind you doubling back and forth below. This is your past life. Up ahead, the way also seems clear. Standing on mental tiptoe, you can see the future.

You now become aware that there are people around you. You feel that the others with whom you travel belong to you. As you glance back down the mountain, you notice people all along the winding path. There are those who are just emerging from the darkness of the valley you left but a short time ago. There is no feeling of superiority, yet you are aware that they cannot see the great distances you can. You bless them on their journey.

You next lift your mental vision to those who are far ahead of you. Their gaze encompasses more than yours, yet there is no feeling of being inferior to them. You know that with a little more climbing, you, too, shall see what they now behold.

With a step that grows lighter the higher you go—with almost a feeling of being lifted up on a cloud—you find yourself standing on a high mesa rim. You are looking out across a vastness, and there seems to be no end to the range of your vision. Because of the height on which you stand, you can encompass what lies before you and behind you in one sweeping view—the BIG VIEW. You can see far back into what was once past. You can peer far ahead into what is future.

You behold the view now with an intense feeling of gratitude for the scope it opens up to you. You study it and soon new impressions and insight take shape. Trends become clear, causes are understood, right courses of action are revealed to you, foresight and retrosight become yours.

You now affirm: *"From this height of consciousness, I feel a new sense of freedom from time. Pressures are gone. Limited understanding is gone. From this height, petty details in the scheme of things fall into place, and the past, present, and future become a comprehensive unit of perception NOW.*

(Close your eyes after reading this several times and mentally dwell in an awareness of the big view you feel. End your HSP-sensitivity session by affirming:)

And so it is!

SUMMARY CAPSULES

RISING ABOVE THE RIVER OF TIME

The real Self of you stands above time on a high plateau of enlightened perception. Far below this real You, there flows with the River of Time a self whose perception is boxed in with daily time-space factors. The purpose of the Science of Higher Sense Perception is to help the time-space you to awaken to this uninvolved, higher, timeless You and its expanded powers.

GAINING POWERS OF FORESIGHT AND RETROSIGHT

As your horizon broadens, you gain the "big view" that extends your awareness into tomorrow and yesterday. You become uncannily sensitive to future trends and past causes. New faculties of foresight and retrosight unfold. Foresight sharpens your judgment and directs you toward success in every endeavor. Retrosight brings empathy and new insight into human motivation.

BREAKING THE TIME-BARRIER TO SUCCESS

Your traditional-time perception is a barrier that limits you to five-sense experiences. This barrier is built by the attention given to the physical and environmental you. To break this barrier, you must give more of your thought and attention to the real You and to the realm of *real cause*. To break free of the pressure and tension of time-oriented thinking, is to enter a new realm of success.

EXPANDING YOUR DIMENSIONAL PERCEPTION

The *average* life revolves in a meager four dimensions of a many-dimensional mental world. Beyond the traditional fourth dimension is a concept of time, a fifth dimension, that pushes out the boundaries of the world you know. To perceive from this higher dimension is to gain an insight that places the past, present, and future in a larger *spacious present*—a timeless fifth dimension.

LIVING WHERE TIME STANDS STILL

In the fifth dimension, the present is the *eternal now*. After all, *now* is the only instant you can be conscious. Now is the only moment you can conceive an idea, create, invent, discover, or contemplate anything. To perform up to your ability in the *eternal now* is to make time stand still. Fears about the future disappear; troubles from the past dissolve! And, you become master of time!

5

How to Use the
Psi-Phone of Telepathy

Can mind meet with mind at a higher level of thought—at a level where time and space are not barriers to communication? Can you use your mind to affect the thinking, feelings, moods, or actions of a person who may be at some distance from you? Finally, can such a faculty be cultivated deliberately?

It can, *unless* you consider that you are a finished product of the evolutionary process with *no* unrefined faculties or latent potentialities. All of nature bears witness to the contrary. Evolution is a *constant* process—a process of ceaseless, restless, eternal unfoldment. This ceaseless urge of life to refine itself has brought man the ability to think, the logic to devise an oral and written language, the capacity to reason, the insight to analyze and synthesize, and the discernment to foresee consequences. Man's conscious equipment seems quite extensive, but from an evolutionary standpoint, his powers are far from complete.

All the faculties man now possesses are capable of further unfoldment, for there is no end to the evolutionary process. His present sensory equipment, expanded, will reveal higher sensory equipment awaiting his use. One such power that even now is emerging is that of telepathy, the extension of man's present faculty of communication.

Telepathy is no myth. It can be used by anyone. In this chapter you will learn how to dial others telepathically and communicate through the universal mental switchboard.

A case of telepathic communication

Marian C. desparately wanted to talk to Van. Something urgent had come up, and she needed his advice. Van was an old friend and someone on whom she could depend. She valued his judgment. However, it was late in the evening and she wasn't sure where he would be. She couldn't call him, for he had moved to a new apartment where the phone was not yet installed. How could she reach him? She felt she simply could not wait until she saw him again.

Now Marian had taken a class I taught on higher sense perception, and she felt that it was possible to make contact with another person telepathically. It suddenly occurred to her that if *she* could not phone Van, perhaps she could get *him* to call her. She had never really needed to use telepathy before. Now she did, and went at it with intense concentration. Acutely motivated by the desire to communicate with him, she began walking back and forth in her room visualizing Van picking up the phone and calling her.

As she paced the floor, she repeated over and over, "Van, call me! This is Marian. I must talk with you. Pick up the phone *now* and call me!" She found herself saying it aloud, and with each exclamation, she pounded her right fist into her cupped left hand. Driving her fist into her hand seemed to make her thoughts more emphatic, and she went on with this intense concentration for perhaps twenty minutes.

Although the phone did not ring and Marian was disappointed, she had worked off enough energy that she was finally able to get to bed and fall asleep.

The following morning, her phone did ring. It was Van calling! Without any prompting regarding the previous evening, he said, "The strangest thing happened last night, Marian. I was sleeping when suddenly I awoke dreaming that you were pounding me on my chest. I sat up with a start, and could still feel where your fists had been beating."

Instantly Marian realized that her telepathic message to Van had come to him symbolically. She told him how she had attempted to reach him, and they checked the time of his dream. It was at the exact moment when she was walking the floor, pounding a fist into her cupped hand, and repeating over and over, "Van, call me!"

A successful experiment in communication

Marian's attempt at telepathy thrilled her. She *did* succeed in establishing rapport with Van. Her thoughts did wake him from a sound sleep, and non-objective communication did take place.

As Marian paced back and forth across the room, driving home her words, her message came through to Van as an inner impression. Because he was asleep, the impression took a symbolic form and registered as the dream that she was pounding him on the chest.

The conclusion is clear that a telepathic message was sent and received, although its reception did not result in the immediate action desired. Van did not awake enough to dress and go out to call Marian at the moment. To her delight, however, he did call her first thing in the morning.

A fascinating point about Marian's experience is that she *dialed* Van after all. True, she did not use an objective telephone, but in HSP terms she used her *psi-phone.* The connection was wireless, of course, and based on their friendship and rapport. Marian used a telepathic principle you are about to discover in this chapter.

The factors that make telepathy possible

The Science of Higher Sense Perception does not simply assert that expanded powers are possible. But, from the first page to the last, scientific facts about the nature of mind are presented that *reveal* expanded powers.

For example, the factors that account for telepathy are revealed in the three-level structure of mind. Those three levels are the conscious (objective mind), subconscious (subjective mind), and superconscious (pure mind.) A form of communication takes place at all three levels.

At the conscious level, you converse objectively with others by means of the spoken or written word, by telephone, by telegraph, by short wave, by television, etc. At the subconscious level, you may converse subjectively with the minds of others via telepathy. At the superconscious level, you may communicate with pure mind by means of intuition.

Psychologists and behavioral scientists have dealt quite extensively with the first two phases of mind—the conscious and the subconscious. Their definitions of these two levels correspond, generally, with the definitions used by the Science of Higher Sense Perception.

Specifically, the *conscious mind* is the reasoning, planning, choosing, analyzing, determining, and initiating mind. The *subconscious* mind is the motor mind that carries out the commands of the conscious—accepting, retaining, creating, serving, and performing. The conscious mind is the thinker; the subconscious is the doer. The conscious mind is the boss; the subconscious mind is the servant. But what a creative and ingenious servant it is!

The conscious and subconscious phases of mind and their reciprocal nature must be understood by every student of Higher Sense Perception. You must know that *consciously* you have the power to decide, choose, and initiate the action you want carried out.

You must also know and appreciate the vast creative ability of the *subconscious,* for it reacts to the action you dictate. In it are contained the motor skills you have developed and the intangible qualities you have acquired. It is the seat of all sensory faculties. It repairs and maintains the body. It is the storehouse of memory. It has infinite know-how. In its functioning it may draw upon all of the known and unknown laws of the universe.

Just because the conscious and subconscious phases of mind have distinct properties does not in any way imply that they are two separate minds. They are simply the two functions of the personal mental equipment you have. Moreover, your personal mental equipment is not strictly *individual.* If it were, there would be no such thing as communication, either objective or subjective! The very fact that two people can communicate means that there must be oneness of mind. This is where the superconscious Mind comes in (the parent Mind common to everyone).

There must be a oneness—a common medium or mode—that makes telepathy possible. It is this same oneness that makes metavision and metaudition possible. It is this oneness that removes the barriers of time and space. The common medium is universal Mind. It is the superconscious. The universal superconscious (pure Mind), individualizing itself as a focal point of conscious awareness, results in man. There, it communicates with separate, individualized points of itself. It communicates *objectively* by means of the spoken or written word. It communicates *subjectively* by such means as telepathy.

The conscious mode of communication

The three levels of mind give rise to the three basic modes of communication you may use to converse with other people and with the world of nature. For, being one with all life, you are in communication with life at all levels whether you realize it or not.

First, there is the conscious-awareness level where you converse with others verbally and visually. This mode utilizes the spoken and written word, pictures, films, images, and symbols, to convey thoughts to others. However, due to semantic gaps in meaning, the language barrier, and ideological blocks to understanding, conscious communication is often inadequate. This inadequacy is spoken of today in one regard as the generation gap.

Man's inability to communicate adequately at the verbal level has led him into war and heartbreak. Too often his meaning and his words are not synchronized. He may say one thing, but mean another. He may be told one thing, but hear another. Man desparately needs to develop true skill in the art of conscious communication.

The telepathic mode of communication

Second, there is a telepathic mode of communication that takes place at the subconscious level. Literally, a degree of telepathic rapport exists between you and others most of the time. The degree may vary in depth and level of intensity. Telepathic rapport ranges from a "first impression" feeling of trust that you may immediately have for another person to a more profound feeling that something has happened to a loved one. It may be a specific instance of telepathic contact such as occured between Marian and Van, or it may be a general feeling of rapport such as man and dog enjoy.

At the subconscious level, you are able to commune with the trees of the forest, with the world beneath your feet, with animals that respond to the feeling states of your mind. My friend, J. Allen Boone, tells in *Kinship with All Life* of the bridge of communication established between himself and Strongheart, the dog who became a celebrity under Boone's tutelage:

> Strongheart broke me of the bad habit of mentally looking down my nose at other living entities and other forms of life as inferior ... Out of this teaching there developed a mental bridge, so to speak, between us. It was a bridge for two-way, not one-directional, thought traffic. With this invisible bridge connecting us, it was possible for my thoughts freely to cross over into his thinking areas and for his thoughts to freely cross over into mine.[1]

The lesson involved here applies to human beings as well as to animals. It is at the subconscious level that mind with mind can meet at a non-verbal, non-objective level of communication. But in order to establish a *bridge of understanding,* mutual respect, empathy, and love are usually essential. When they exist, profound experiences in telepathic rapport may occur. Such was the case with Ruth P.

A case study of telepathic rapport

A feeling of uneasiness persisted for Ruth P. all morning. Something was wrong, but what? Ruth had made a study of telepathy and had developed considerable ability in using higher powers of mind. She had felt this characteristic uneasiness before, so she tried to relax and let the message manifest.

She went about her housework routinely, keeping her mind in a listening mood. Noon came and she prepared lunch, eating it without much relish. She was washing dishes when there flashed upon the screen of her mind a picture of her mother on a stretcher. The stretcher was being raised into an ambulance. She saw her father and sister standing by watching the ambulance drive away. Then, the scene was gone!

After the telepathic flash, which came in visual form, Ruth collected herself and put through a long distance call to her parents' home. Ruth lived in Colorado. Her parents and sister were

———————
1
Boone, J. Allen, *Kinship With All Life.* New York: Harper & Row, Publishers, Inc., 1954, p. 74.

residing in Florida. Her sister, Ann, answered the phone. Normally, Ann would not have been there, but Ruth *knew* who would answer. She asked Ann the extent of the heart attack which her mother had just suffered. Ann was astonished, "You mean you already know! Why, the ambulance left only a short time ago, and we don't know yet the seriousness of the attack."

After talking to Ann, Ruth put in a call to the hospital. Somehow she *knew* her mother would be in the local hospital in the small town where she lived and not at a large city hospital near by. She talked to the doctor in charge, and he told her that it was too early to be definite but that her mother was responding as well as could be expected.

Ruth called Ann back to tell her of the conversation with the doctor. Here was Ruth, two thousand miles from the scene, telling her sister, who was less than three miles from the hospital, of the condition of their mother.

This example clearly shows that at HSP levels of awareness, the distance that exists at the physical level is not a relevant factor. At the higher reaches of awareness, the concept of *near* and *far* lose their significance and no longer restrict man's sense perception.

How to attune to telepathic messages

The message Ruth received of her mother's attack came through as clearly as a telephone call. She "saw" part of it; she interiorly "knew" part of it. Who was responsible for sending the message? Who was responsible for receiving it?

Was the sender Ruth's mother or some other member of the family who thought of Ruth in that moment of crisis? It is impossible to say, because most instances of telepathy originate at the subjective level and are not conscious acts of the sender.

Thomas Jay Hudson, long an authority on psychic phenomena, affirms that telepathy is typically a subconscious activity:

> Telepathy is the means of communion between subjective minds. The objective mind does not necessarily participate in the communication. The message, in other words, is not necessarily on a subject of which either party is consciously thinking. It frequently has no connection whatever with the conscious thoughts of either of the participants in the production of the phenomena.[2]

---

[2]Hudson, Thomas Jay, *A Scientific Demonstration of the Future Life.* Chicago: A. C. McClurg and Company, 1895, p. 68.

This seems to be true in Ruth's case. The message probably had no connection with the *conscious* thoughts of the participants. However, when the feeling of uneasiness came to Ruth, she cooperated consciously by putting herself in a receptive state. She attuned herself by relaxing and assuming a "listening" attitude. Hence, she *was* responsible for receiving the message.

The uneasy feeling Ruth experienced is characteristic of the apprehension that often precedes reception of telepathic, clair-voyant, and other HSP messages. You may wonder what to do at such a time.

If you wish to consciously cooperate and attune to such messages, use the Psi-Programmer below. Its purpose is to help you relax by dissolving the apprehension and anxiety that may accompany pre-telepathic message reception. A listening attitude is difficult to maintain if you are fearful that you may tune into negative news.

Therefore, program protection for yourself into your "listening" attitude by affirming that no message received will harm you or shock you. Affirm that whatever is received can come through only in a form which will be for your total good.

Ψ   Psi-Programming Pointer
AS NONCHALANTLY AS I ANSWER THE PHONE AND LISTEN, I NOW LISTEN FOR THE VOICE OF TELEPATHY. ITS MESSAGE IS FOR MY TOTAL GOOD AND LEAVES ME UNWORRIED AND UNAFRAID.

The intuitive mode of higher communication

Above and beyond the type of communication Van and Ruth received—which took place at the subjective level—there is a third mode of communication. This is direct communication with superconscious Mind. Here the individual does not simply use universal Mind as a medium through which messages are communicated from one mind to another, but he contacts the ultimate source of Mind directly and intimately. This contact brings a feeling of insight and inspiration. It is *intuition*—the awareness of pure knowledge.

Communion with pure Mind is the way of the mystic, not the way of the psychic. In Chapter 6, a detailed explanation of the difference between the mystic and the psychic is given.

What you need to recognize *now* is that while individual minds can tune into each other telepathically, the individual can also tune into higher levels of mind. Telepathy and the powers that await man on the subconscious level are vast, it is true. But the source from which these powers flow is vaster still. This source is the third and ultimate level of mind—the superconscious. Superconscious Mind (universal Mind) is the *universality* which gives rise to all individuality. Individually, you are universality individualized.

To recapitulate briefly, at the conscious level of mind, you converse with others verbally and visually. At the subconscious depths, you may telepathically commune with the minds of others. At the higher superconscious level, you may intuitively perceive the more interior truths resident in pure Mind. Here intuition may manifest as the *still, small voice* of sacred literature.

To help you utilize mind better at all three levels—the conscious, the subconscious, and superconscious—is the purpose of the Science of Higher Sense Perception.

Tuning into the telepathic frequencies of others

Telepathy, as well as other psi-abilities, cannot be understood or fully appreciated until it is recognized that man is not a body—not a physical house. Man is the mental being who lives *in* the House-of-Self. That mental being is a composite—a blend—of the unique experiences and attitudes that make up his consciousness.

That composite exists as a rate of vibration. Comparing it to electricity, it could be called a frequency. The closer your consciousness approaches the frequency of another person's consciousness, the more rapport you will experience.

You have had the surprise of tuning into the thoughts of others many times. You may have been thinking of someone only to have him call you on the telephone or see him at the door a moment later. Or perhaps a letter arrived from a friend evoking from you the exclamation, "Why, I was just thinking of him yesterday."

Because of a closeness in consciousness (a rapport) you both were in tune. Perhaps that rapport was a common interest, or a common problem, or a common affection for each other.

This same rapport takes place at a more universal level with the great in every field who are able to communicate to you their artistry and rhythm. A great poet communicates through the beauty of the written word. A fine musician communicates through the cosmic harmony of his music. A skilled painter expresses through the medium of his art.

However, the artistry of the poet or musician or painter will not be communicated to the individual who has nothing in his consciousness that is *in tune.* The closer you are in consciousness to the frequency on which another person vibrates, the better will be the communication. If someone "turns you on," you are communicating—you are vibrating on the same frequency of consciousness.

Similarly, telepathy may occur when two minds are tuned to the same frequency. Mental rapport establishes a line of communication above the level of conscious, verbal interchange. It is like two or more minds striking a mental high "C" in unison.

Using the universal mental switchboard

The dictionary definition of *telepathy* is *"apparent communication from one mind to another otherwise than through the channels of sense; thought transference."* Telepathy is usually considered to be a phenomenon that involves individual mind with individual mind. But telepathy also has a broad aspect which must not be ignored. It is true that one person may communicate with another person, either verbally or by means of thought, but the level of your consciousness also connects you with a related level of universal consciousness.

It might be said that the mental universe is a vast switchboard panel relaying messages to receivers who are in rapport. Messages of a negative character are received by those who deliberately or inadvertently converse in like tones with others. Hence, a negative consciousness connects you with negative circuits on the universal mental switchboard. Conversely, a consciousness of success plugs you into a success circuit. Just as the town gossip attracts to her all those on the party line who have rumors to spread, so the negative individual attracts to himself others who have negation to spread.

You can discriminately choose the messages that are relayed to you through the universal switchboard by disciplining your own consciousness. With psi-training techniques, you can alter your consciousness and make it more constructive and positive. New positive attitudes will bring you into rapport with those who are creative and successful.

If you are pessimistic, you will inadvertently "dial" whatever elements of pessimism another person entertains. However, if you are optimistic, you will ring up elements of optimism latent in others.

Telepathy as a factor in demonstrating success

Once you know that rapport and communication are established between you and those who are close to you in consciousness, it would be folly to sustain a consciousness of self-defeat, pessimism, and failure. Rather, you must deliberately entertain mental images of success and affluence. Such thoughts will put you in rapport with success elements in the consciousness of those with whom you deal.

Want to dial into success circuits in your particular field? Then make your mental state positive, as did Matt J.

Matt, a struggling insurance agent, heard a lecture I gave on the universal mental switchboard. He grasped at once that he had been tuning into failure circuits. "Why, with every prospect who turned me down, my fear of failure grew worse. It's a wonder I sold any insurance at all!"

"And now?" I prodded.

"Now it's just like I am guided to the right propsect at the right time. Almost without exception," Matt exclaimed, "those I call on are in the market for a policy, and I just happen along to serve their needs."

"But it is no *chance* happening!"

"True," Matt agreed. "Now I deliberately dial into success circuits by filling my mind with attitudes of success. As you suggested, I sit down in quiet contemplation and visualize contacts with prospects who really need the type of policy I can give them. I actually *feel* the joy and satisfaction of serving people well. I *feel* the thrill of their appreciation. I *make* my mental state positive."

"Only after this mental work," Matt continued, "do I make actual phone calls or office visits. I limit those calls to the names I feel good about. And, it really works! I seem to be in special telepathic rapport with the prospects I call. It's almost as if they expected me!"

Because like attracts like, when Matt raised his mental state to a success-level, he attuned himself to the success-level of others. He "dialed" a circuit on the universal switchboard that resulted in happy communication for all concerned. You can do the same for yourself by conditioning your thoughts with the Psi-Programming Pointer below.

Ψ   Psi-Programming Pointer
I NOW CREATE A POSITIVE MENTAL STATE. THAT
STATE ATTUNES ME TO SUCCESS CIRCUITS ON THE
UNIVERSAL MENTAL SWITCHBOARD AND CONNECTS ME
WITH OTHERS AT A SUCCESS-LEVEL.

How to turn black magic into white magic

The use to which Matt put his telepathic psi-ability is not coercion, will power, or black magic. It is the use of an individual's freedom to dial others at their success-level. If your desires and intentions harmonize with the well being of another, rapport will be established and blessings will result for both of you in telepathic interchange. Otherwise, no rapport will occur.

Of course, instances have occurred where, through sheer will power, mental manipulation, or so-called black magic, apparent harm has been inflicted by one person upon another. This can never happen when your telepathic psi-contact with another is governed by the stipulation that results are for the benefit of all concerned.

The main power behind black magic is the credulity of both parties involved. *Black magic* is defined as *"an irresistible influence or fascination; enchantment."* It is the use of mental power in reverse. It is an enchantment with the negative instead of the positive. Certainly, those who are attuned to negative messages from the universal switchboard experience that which is black and bleak.

Black magic is popularly associated with voodoo practices such as the attempt to harm an enemy by sticking pins into a small effigy of him. It is conceivable that if an enemy *believed* in such mental influence he would experience its effects.

A subtler type of black magic is practiced by those who attempt by undue influence and will power to sell worthless stocks and promote fly-by-night schemes. The power of mind can be used to control others, but a negative use of psi-ability will not lead to success. It may lead to a sale, but its practice will result in eventual disaster, not success.

The positive use of your higher-sense-perception powers may appropriately be called *white magic.* White magic is the use of your mental powers for the benefit and blessing of all with whom you deal. You go, and grow, to greatness through a recognition of good for yourself and others. Dial that universal level of consciousness which is constructive and positive! As you do so, you will be guided telepathically to others with like thoughts. You will, in turn, be "dialed" by those who wish you well, who desire for you the highest and best that life has to offer.

Black magic is to exert control for selfish reasons; white magic is to hold others in a selfless mental embrace of good will and understanding.

How to dial the psi-phone of good will

Just as you are able to pick up the telephone and dial the number of a friend and receive an answer, so you are able to dial the psi-phone of others with whom you are in rapport.

In psychology, it is recognized that rapport is often experienced by twins, by sisters, and by parents and their offspring. The explanation for this phenomenon has been sought in heredity. But, the true explanation is not physical; it is psychical. Those who are close to one another are subconsciously connected by the psi-phone of common purpose and understanding. Usually, they share a love, a feeling of concern, a desire for the well-being of each other and a mutual respect that obliterates any feeling of "superiority" or "inferiority." This constitutes mental rapport.

Remember what J. Allen Boone learned from his movie-dog friend, Strongheart. He found that Stronghheart did not like the feeling that his human was looking down his nose at him. Communication has to be on a like frequency. You can't go through life looking down on dogs—or on people—as inferior. Just as Strongheart knocked the nonsense of superiority out of Boone's head, you must rid your head of such nonsense when dealing with your fellowman.

Consider the meaning of *communication.* To communicate does not mean, "listen to me!" It means *"to commune, to confer together, to converse intimately."* Many personal problems, as well as world problems, are due to a superiority feeling—the feeling that cooperation means, "Listen to what I say!" Communication must be a two-way street. It must involve two-way thought traffic. There must be talking and listening and understanding.

To demonstrate rapport with another you must establish the two-way thought traffic of understanding. You must speak on the horizontal and listen on the horizontal. Bring your life into alignment with the lives of others through a recognition of your oneness with the one Mind that is the cause of all. This recognition will synchronize your life with universal Mind and enable you to tune into the thought frequencies of more and more people.

Because Marian and Van were attuned to each other, she was able to make *specific* contact with him. Because Matt attuned himself to a success circuit, he was able to make *general* contact with others at their success-level. In their own ways, they applied the telepathic psi-phone principles explained in this chapter and now summarized for your use:

First. In your mind's eye, go into your House-of-Self—deep into the interior of your being. Here, visualize a telephone. It is a unique phone. Although wireless, its circuits extend infinitely in all directions. It is your *psi-phone.*

Second. In your imagination, picture a telephone book beside your psi-phone. It is a curious book. It contains only the numb of those with whom you are in rapport. The potentiality of communication is best with people with whom you enjoy mutual interest, common purpose, respect, and good will. Missing from your book are the numbers of anyone with whom communication would not be a blessing.

Third. In your mind's eye, look at the dial of your telepathic psi-phone. There are no numbers, just letters—and only four. The letters are L-O-V-E. The meaning of the four is utterly clear. It is through their use that positive rapport may be established in the practice of telepathy.

Fourth. Remember how emphatic Marian was with the message she wished to communicate? In using the psi-phone training technique that follows, make your message brief, concise, and emphatic. Be certain that the intent of the message is constructive and worth while; then convey it with urgency and emphasis!

HSP-SENSITIVITY TRAINING TECHNIQUE NO. 5

DIALING YOUR TELEPATHIC PSI-PHONE

You are seated in your favorite chair. You relax, breathe deeply, and read this over until you can follow it mentally. Then, you close your eyes and imagine yourself to be deep within your own House-of-Self. Out of the interior darkness before you emerges the outline of a telephone. Its shape is formed of a shimmering silvery light. You note that rays from the light seem to extend infinitely in all directions.

Your gaze remains fixed on the image of the phone before you. It is your psi-phone. You know that it is symbolic of your telepathic ability to contact anyone with whom you are in harmony.

You now plan your call, identifying the specific good which is to result from the contact—an outcome that is for the mutual benefit and blessing of all concerned.

In your mind's eye you now reach out and pick up the receiver. You realize that to make your call you must draw close in consciousness to the frequency on which the person you are calling vibrates. You must connect through *rapport*. Your eye falls on the four-letter dial: L-O-V-E. Only through its use can positive rapport be established. You, therefore, take these steps:

Step 1-"L"-Listen Quietly

"L"-You listen quietly to the heartbeat of the universe. You and your fellowman are one with it. It is the one pulse-of-life that beats within you both. Hear it? It is the dial-tone hum of your psi-phone.

Step 2-"O"-Open the Circuit

"O"-You open the circuit by dismissing mental and emotional blocks. You feel no envy, no criticism, no antagonism, no ill will. Only good will exists between you and the person you wish to contact.

Step 3-"V"-Verify Value

"V"-You verify the value of your message. You affirm its positive purpose. You invoke protection and guidance for yourself by declaring that good, and good alone, is all that can result for those involved.

Step 4-"E"-Emphatically Express

"E"-You emphatically express the specific message you wish to convey, making it concise, brief, and urgent.

You sit quietly and you dial your psi-phone by contemplating the steps that L-O-V-E spell. The dial-tone changes to a ring, and you are suddenly aware that your *feeling of oneness* is ringing up the consciousness of the one you are calling.

Your telepathic psi-call tells him of your good will, and it brings his good will as a response. In your mind's eye, you see him hearing and understanding your message. You visualize him acting upon it and benefitting from it. The call results in mutual good for you both.

You sit quietly for a time after you feel contact has been made, stepping gradually out of the feeling of rapport you have experienced. Then, relax, rejoice, and declare:

And so it is!

SUMMARY CAPSULES

HOW SYNCHRONIZATION MAKES TELEPATHY WORK

To tune into the thoughts of another telepathically, it is necessary to synchronize with his consciousness. Mentally, a harmonious state of thought and feeling must exist, uniting on an interior level sensitized by love, regard, empathy, and oneness of interest. Synchronization implies an interest in the well-being of another that interlocks with your own, at least temporarily. For the moment, rapport is established and telepathy is possible.

WHAT A HARMONIOUS FREQUENCY DOES

Each person is a sending and receiving station of thought power, but each operates on his own unique mental frequency. The invisible lines of communication broadcast constantly from your mind find reception in the mind of others attuned to your station. Your mental frequency, if negative, attracts those who vibrate at negative levels. How important it is that you keep your tone of consciousness at a high positive level of success!

WHAT TWO-WAY TRAFFIC OF UNDERSTANDING MEANS

To communicate with life successfully, you must develop two-way thought traffic. You cannot look down your nose at other people or at other forms of life, considering them inferior. Other human beings and other creatures are different from you, but they are neither inferior nor superior. They are simply different. Two-way thought traffic is established with them as you converse on an even level of understanding without downgrading their status.

HOW TO DIAL YOUR TELEPATHIC PSI-PHONE

To successfully dial your psi-phone and communicate a consciousness of understanding, love, peace, and well-being to another, you must select the number belonging to the good you desire. You cannot dial the number for fear and expect faith or dial hate and expect good will to answer. Love responds to the code number for it alone. Keep your psi-phone call one of high regard, of lofty intentions, and of sincere concern for yourself and others.

HOW TO TAP UPPER REACHES OF COMMUNICATION

At the conscious level you converse with the minds of others verbally and visually. On the subconscious plane, you may communicate with the minds of others telepathically. At the superconscious level, you are able to commune with pure Mind. Here, on this upper plane, is the origin of all knowledge, all laws, all principles. By an intuitive process—the process of the mystic—you may tap superconscious Mind and perceive the interior truths of life.

6

How to Tap the Psychic
and the Mystic Levels

There was no mistake about it—the lady was going to have a
KADALAK. At least, this is what the Ouija board said.

The group that had gathered for an evening of fun were
clustered around two women who sat facing each other. Their
attention was riveted on an oblong board supported like a table by
their knees. Their fingers rested lightly on a tear-shaped disk that
glided across the board on three tiny felt-tipped legs. A hush had
fallen over the group as one of the two women asked, "Ouija,
what kind of a car will my husband buy when we trade in our old
one?"

In the silence of the room, the disk began to move beneath their
fingers. At first it seemed that one of the two participants must be
pushing the pointed disk, but it moved so fast—deftly maneuvering
back and forth and turning around under their fingers—that it was
obviously self-impelled. All eyes were intent upon it as it moved
toward the alphabet letters on the board. It pointed first to the K,
next to the A, then to the D, back again to the A, then to L, A,
and K.

"Why, I think it's trying to spell Cadillac," Flo, the older of the
two participants, exclaimed. "Let's check one more time!" Again
the question was asked, and the Ouija pointer uncannily moved
across the board, faithfully spelling again K-A-D-A-L-A-K.

"Well," laughed one in the group gathered around the board, "If Ouija means a Cadillac, it certainly is ignorant when it comes to spelling."

The party wore on, and other questions were asked. The Ouija pointer moved to and fro, sometimes answering with comprehensible words, sometimes with jibberish. Finally the pointer turned stubbornly to the word GOODBYE printed at the bottom of the board, and the Ouija set was put away. The party broke up, and the guests went their separate ways. They'd had a good time, and no one took Ouija's messages seriously. The incident of the KADALAK was pushed to the back of Flo's mind, and she almost forgot it. The possibility of her husband buying a Cadillac seemed far-fetched, and she dismissed the idea.

Flo's husband was a skillful business man. The real estate company he had built up from nothing was beginning to prosper. In fact, he was doing much better than Flo realized. It had been his nature to be good to himself, and he permitted himself a luxury or two whenever he could afford it.

It was not too long after the party that Flo's husband began talking about buying a new car. He shopped around for a while, looking at one make after another. Then, one evening, he calmly announced that he had ordered a new Cadillac.

Flo was astonished. "You mean we can afford one?"

Her husband quieted her, explaining, "It will be a good investment."

Flo suddenly remembered Ouija's prophecy! How did the Ouija know their new car would be a KADALAK?

How is a Ouija Board message explained?

How is such a message to be explained? Does some valid principle underlie the Ouija-board phenomenon or is it merely a toy? Of course, the phenomenon can always be called a coincidence. But, what is a coincidence?

A dictionary defines *coincidence* as, *1. The condition or fact of an instance of coinciding; correspondence; 2. A group of concurrent events or circumstances remarkable for lack of apparent causal connection.* How does that grab you? Now, do you know what a coincidence is?

Labeling something a coincidence is a convenient device for dismissing it without bothering to search for a cause. There may be *a lack of apparent cause,* but what about hidden, unseen causes? These are the causes that must be probed.

The purpose of this chapter is to uncover the non-apparent laws that operate behind the objective scene—laws that account for psychic and mystic phenomena. In the pages that follow, you will discover the kind of action that may occur on the *lower psychic level,* often referred to as the psychic sea. Above this lies the *higher psychic level* where you can utilize extended mind principles to demonstrate HSP powers that are reliable. Finally, you will be introduced to the kind of phenomenon that takes place at the mystic level. You will learn what laws the psychic works with at the subconscious level and what upper reaches the mystic knows at the superconscious level.

What is the so-called psychic sea?

The real things of life are unseen. You do not see mind, ideas, motives, attitudes, or feelings. What you see are the effects brought about by these causes. Once the effect is produced, does the cause cease to be? Does the idea in the mind of an inventor cease to exist on the unseen plane just because his invention is produced and marketed? Does the mathematical concept in the mind of an Einstein cease to be after it is put down on paper? In fact, does any idea cease to be once it is expressed? Do the astral impressions left by the passage of any event really cease to be? No, from all evidence, it appears that ideas and impressions tend to persist. They tend to become part of the thought atmosphere in which mankind lives, and moves, and has its being. This collective atmosphere, subconscious in nature, has been called the psychic record or the psychic sea.

Each individual, through the ages, has contributed to this collective atmosphere from his own individual consciousness. This collective consciousness is now the subjective sea which surrounds man. It is like the ocean that surrounds the fish as it swims or the air that surrounds the bird as it flies.

What is the nature of the lower psychic level?

This subjective psychic atmosphere is not unlike the blanket of air that surrounds the earth. Within that aerial envelope move great wind currents and the trade-winds of the oceans. Massive cold currents of air flowing from the polar regions replace the warmer and lighter air ascending from the tropical belt to create complex and challenging conditions. No less challenging are the *psychic currents of mind.*

Negative currents of thought have been generated in the psychic atmosphere through the ages by those who espouse greed and ruthlessness. Great counter currents of good have been created by humanitarians who value the basic worth and rights of the individual. The cross-currents that result from the interaction of these psychic winds keep the world in turmoil.

The well-being of society, the establishment of peace between the peoples of the world, and the maintenance of personal happiness are to be found in the psychic currents that mankind chooses to follow.

Aside from the great psychic streams of consciousness which are comparable to the global winds of our planet, there are also local atmospheric conditions to consider in understanding the nature of the lower psychic level. The collective thinking of mankind creates a thought-envelope as real as the smog-envelope that has surrounded many a city. Immediately surrounding you is the thought-content emanating from your own and other contemporary minds. Visualize those who populate your world as smokestacks of various height and size. Like the smokestacks that dot the skyline of an industrial town, each is emitting a vapor of a different color and intensity. Some emissions may be benign and harmless. Some may be irritating, obnoxious, and injurious. Collectively, they form the mental atmosphere of the *lower psychic level.*

It must be stressed how *diverse* the mental elements are that go into the makeup of the lower psychic level. Vagrant wishes and desires may form a part of it. The impressions left by events that have transpired and events that are in the making are part of it.

Mass anxieties and fears may color it. Creative and inventive ideas may slip into it. The lower psychic level is the *mixing bowl of mind* just beyond the conscious level. It is the level from which you get moods and impressions. The level from which you may pick up unexplained anxieties. Information from it may or may not be reliable, for it is a jumble of mental elements.

This is the *mental-smog level,* where some information is relatively pure but where much is the waste product of poorly processed thinking.

"Ouija, speak to me . . . "

This is the level at which Ouija spoke to Flo. Of the many messages the two women spelled out that night at the party, this was the only one which proved to be true. A Ouija board speaks from the mental-smog level where it is difficult to distinguish between truths, half-truths, and error. Nevertheless, Ouija did answer this question correctly! What, then, is the explanation?

This is the question Flo asked me as I chatted with a group of HSP students at class one evening. She had just told us her story of the KADALAK, and now she asked me, "How did Ouija know?"

A class member broke in half jokingly, "Flo, maybe you have an unseen Indian guide who spoke through Ouija!"

I hastened to add, "That's a theory shared by some, but let's examine another explanation. Flo, let me put it this way: Ouija can't know anything you don't know."

"But," Flo objected adamantly, "I had *no* idea my husband could afford a Cadillac!"

"Of course, you had no *conscious* idea, but what about the knowledge that comes through the subconscious? You see, all of us are in possession of greater wisdom than we consciously know. The knowledge you have access to at the conscious level is minute compared with the data-resources of the subconscious. Much information which the individual has, but of which he is not consciously aware, can be lifted from the subconscious to the conscious level through a sincere desire to know. It may come through a simple toy-like device such as a Ouija board, or it may come through deep meditation, or dreams."

"You mean," Flo asserted, "that I knew subconsciously that we were going to buy a Cadillac?"

"Not necessarily, but your subconscious may have picked up an idea communicated to the psychic record by your husband. Flo, tell me what your husband was like."

"Well, he was very secretive for one thing. And, he was in the habit of treating himself very well. He always bought himself the finest suits. He kept me in the dark about his income, but I always suspected he was doing better than he'd admit. You know," Flo declared, "I'll bet he had planned secretly to get a Cadillac for a long time!"

"Subconsciously, then, you picked up information that was in the psychic record. You see, although you directed your request to 'Ouija,' you were really tapping the psychic record through your subconscious mind. This can happen when you are sincere and receptive—not just asking in jest."

"But," Flo wondered, "why was the spelling of Cadillac so illiterate?"

"Was it, really? Sounding out K-A-D-A-L-A-K, it is phonetically accurate and is in keeping with the symbolic language in which the subconscious so often speaks. The subconscious uses this same type of symbolism in dreams."

"I can understand that," Flo replied, "but what made the Ouija pointer move. I certainly didn't push it!"

"Telekinetic energy is responsible for phenomenon like that. Your own mind-power is capable of projecting itself as a physical force beyond the confines of the body. You provided the Ouija board and your subconscious mind provided the telekinetic energy to move the pointer and bring you the message."

Flo's experience was dramatic. It illustrates the kind of action that may take place at the lower psychic level. However, it should encourage no one to dabble in the psychic record for reliable direction. For, there is no way to distinguish between fact and wishful thinking or to separate sense from nonsense at this level (unless a guidance command is programmed into the subconscious to screen out half-truths.)

The phenomenon of automatic writing

Another kind of action that may be experienced at the lower psychic level is automatism—automatic writing. Here a person who is able to relax the conscious mind may find that he can hold a pencil in his hand and, without conscious direction, let the subconscious express on the paper before him. Much of what is written may be unintelligible, especially at the beginning. As the technique is practiced more, meaningful material may come forth. It must be remembered that the subconscious has access to data long forgotten consciously. It has access through the psychic record to the thoughts of great minds down through the ages.

Jim, another member of the class, was fascinated by the mention of automatic writing. I explained that it is a device for letting the subconscious mind speak and is similar to Ouija board phenomena. When you are in a receptive state, the subconscious mind may tap data in the psychic record and transmit it to you through non-directed hand movements. Your own subconscious provides the telekinetic energy to move the pencil.

"Can we do it?" Jim asked. A number of other class members were eager to try, also.

"Well," I said, "automatic writing can be cultivated, and you may wish to try it as an experiment in probing the powers of the subconscious."

First, relax comfortably with a pad of paper on your lap and a ball-point pen resting poised for use in your hand.

Second, assume a quiet, contemplative state, still the conscious mind, blank out all exterior thoughts, and concentrate solely on the words of the Psi-Programming Pointer below. Repeat it slowly, over and over.

Third, as you repeat the psi-programmer, let your hand move aimlessly, without deliberate direction, over the paper. At first, much of what is written or drawn will be akin to doodling. It may seem to be mere jibberish. However, as more receptivity develops and more reliance is placed on the subconscious, meaningful material may come forth. It may be long-forgotten material from the deeper recesses of your mind or material from the psychic record.

Ψ   Psi-Programming Pointer
MY MOVING HAND NOW SPEAKS TO ME OF KNOW-
LEDGE AND WISDOM FROM THE SUBCONSCIOUS, KNOW-
LEDGE THAT ENHANCES MY ABILITY AND PROMOTES
MY WELL-BEING.

Precautions in the practice of automatism

"Is there any danger in developing automatic writing?" Jim wanted to know.

I emphasized that those who wanted to try it should not regard it too lightly.

First, don't assume that everything which comes to you through automatic writing is original. Unintentional instances of plagiarism have resulted from picking up creative material from other minds through the subconscious. Sometimes automatic writing has a curious Shakespearean flavor or sounds suspiciously like Hemingway.

However, do not be afraid to express yourself for fear that another person may have tuned into the idea ahead of you. Rather, busy yourself with bringing forth creative ideas before someone else capitalizes on them and grabs the glory.

Second, don't relinquish to subconscious control your prerogative as conscious director without programming into mind the command that you can regain conscious control whenever you wish. Don't allow the subconscious to usurp control. It has been known to happen.

For example, a prominent physician found that he was able to write automatically and practiced the art for a time. Then, one day while with a patient, he was bewildered to find his hand uncontrollably lifted shoulder high while his fingers wrote mechanically in the air.

In chapter Ten you will find specific programming techniques for using subconscious power but retaining, always, the prerogative of conscious control—control that the above doctor lost temporarily. Moreover, you will find that the training techniques given in the Science of Higher Sense Perception are directed toward the *expansion* of the conscious mind and not toward the relinquishment of it to the subconscious.

The phenomenon of automatism in other areas

The phenomenon of automatism—involuntary subconscious control—may also manifest in the field of art or music as automatic painting or playing. But, perhaps the most dramatic manifestation of the phenomenon is in automatic speaking. In its more intense expression, it is called glossalallia or *speaking in tongues.*

It occurs most commonly as part of the devotional experience of various emotion-packed religious groups. As the intensity of a prayer meeting grows, a certain member of the group may be gripped with an uncontrollable urge to speak out. The words are strange and foreign to the ear.

As a child, I attended a church where speaking in tongues was a common practice. There was no fakery involved, for these people were my friends and neighbors, and their honesty was unquestioned. Many were very sincere and beautiful souls, always willing to help where needed. However, they were not aware of what was really happening.

I submit that their *speaking in tongues* was a form of automatism. At highly-charged moments, the emotional center may usurp control of the body. The conscious mind temporarily relinquishes its directional role, and the emotional, which is a *sub*-conscious center, takes over to direct the speech.

This still leaves the question: What explains the strange tongue that is spoken? Is it actually a foreign language or just unintelligible jibberish from the subconscious? As a matter of speculation, assume for a moment that reincarnation is a fact—that the individual has lived before in a different age and culture. Perhaps he spoke an ancient language, no remnants of which remain today. However, in the deep recesses of the *subconscious memory-bank,* the ancient tongue may still persist. Conceivably, then, this lost language may re-express during times of involuntary speaking.

The strange words uttered in the phenomenon of glossalallia, hence, might possibly stem from a long-lost language. Or, the strange utterances may stem from some abnormal state of emotional excitement and frenzy. Or, the phenomenon may simply arise from an intensification of man's normal state of mind!

To clarify, look at man in what is called his normal state. Is he always 100 percent conscious of what he is saying? Is he completly logical, reasonable, and rational in the words he utters? Or, do his words frequently spring from the subconscious, accounting for the things he blurts out uncontrollably?

You have heard the expression, "I could just bite my tongue off for saying that!" People are not as consciously in control of their tongues as they would like to believe. Many, who have never heard of speaking in tongues, let themselves become automatic speakers—echo speakers mouthing over and over again old gripes, animosities, prejudices, distortions, superstitions and rumors stored away in the subconscious.

Many let their tongues wag in one direction while they purport to go in another. This, too, is actually a form of automatism. The person who gossips on and on with little conscious thought is a compulsive speaker. In its way, compulsive speaking is a form of relinquishment of control to the subconscious. In an intensified, emotional form, it may account for much that is called glossalallia.

Difference between automatism and inspiration

Inspirational writing and speaking differ considerably from the automatic kind. Automatic writing and speaking are subjective. They are phenomena associated with the lower psychic level where that which has already been written, spoken, experienced, or thought may be tapped subconsciously. This is the realm of the psychic.

On the other hand, inspirational expression—in fields such as poetry, music, and literature—is a phenomenon associated with the superconscious level. At this higher level, man goes not to the psychic record of what *has been* or *now is,* but he goes to the potential of all that *may be.* At the superconscious level, he deals with pure principles of mind—the raw material—from which new creations result. This is the realm of the mystic.

However, let it be noted here that there are no clear-cut boundaries between the various levels of consciousness. They merge like the air layers above the earth. Earlier in the chapter, the psychic atmosphere surrounding man was compared to the discolored, particle-filled air hovering over a city. Think of this as the *lower psychic level.*

Just above this smog-envelope, the air becomes clear and you can see great distances. Think of this as the *higher psychic level* where expanded perception is possible and the psychic may experience metavision, metaudition, telepathy, etc.

Still higher is the rarified atmosphere where none of the pollution of the earth extends. Think of this as the *mystic level,* the pure level of mind into which man can ascend in consciousness. Here is where inspiration is possible and the mystic may experience intuition—the instant knowledge that derives from tapping pure principle.

It would be foolish to try to locate a point where psychic perception ends and mystic intuition begins. There is a difference, but higher sense perception blends upward into mystical experience. Many notable speakers and writers have utilzed both of these levels—the perceptive and the intuitive—to overcome the cold, sterile style of conscious-effort writing.

William Blake, the artist-poet, has often been cited as one who perceived from the subjective level as well as from the higher mystic plane. In his biography, he is described as "a man whose vivid and eccentric imagination found expression in his mystical poetry and his illustrations for it. For him, heaven, earth, and hell were continuous and contiguous areas through which his mind moved with ease and a feeling of reality."[1]

Not only great writers, but men of genius of all ages and in all fields, have tapped the inspirational level of mind and have utilized it, often in an almost compulsive way. Automatism, too, has been an avenue through which great writers have gathered together thoughts that have enriched our literature.

Harriet A. Boswell, in *Master Guide to Psychism,* says:

> Inspirational work is done with complete awareness of what is to be done next. The idea comes for a melody, painting, or literary work. It is heard or seen in its complete likeness, as a rule . . . Inspirational work has contributed much to the beauty of our world, as most people realize. What is not understood is that automatism has done its share also. In the field of literature, there are many well-known authors who are believed to have received much, if not all, of their works automatically. Two of the best known are Victor Hugo and Goethe.[2]

The Psychic and the Mystic defined

The psychic deals with knowledge that comes to him through the route of the subconscious. It is knowledge already *on record—*

---

[1] Wallace, Helen Kingsbury, *The Encyclopedia Americana.* New York: Grolier, Incorporated, 1956, Vol. IV, p. 57.

[2] Boswell, Harriet A., *Master Guide to Psychism.* New York: Parker Publishing Co., 1969, p. 102.

i.e., it is the perception of what *has* happened, what *is* happening, or what *shall* happen (based on present trends).

When the psychic permits the subconscious to assume a dominant role with little conscious direction, he is working at the *lower psychic level.* The subconscious is not discriminating, unless directed. Hence, results received under these conditions may not be reliable or desirable. Here the psychic is simply wading about aimlessly in the psychic sea of impressions.

However, when the psychic retains conscious control and directs the subconscious toward specific, constructive ends, tremendous realms of perception open up. Results at this level are reliable and rewarding, for the subconscious mind will accomplish with obedient ingenuity the job it is commanded to perform. This is the *higher psychic level,* the realm of HSP.

To summarize briefly: *The lower psychic level involves the relinquishment of conscious direction to the subconscious. The higher psychic level involves expanded conscious direction of subconscious power.*

The mystic, by contrast, deals not with knowledge of this thing or that. Rather, he deals with the raw materials from which knowledge is derived. This is the realm of pure principle or truth. Mystical experience takes place at the superconscious level and arises out of union with the Life principle. The dictionary defines *mystical experience* as an awareness *"relating to, or resulting from, an individual's communion with God or Ultimate Reality."*

This is a valid definition. It indicates that the mystic contacts First Cause—the ultimate or original reality—from which all else results. Through intuition, the mystic becomes aware of a principle. Let's say it is the principle of harmony resident in First Cause. He is so completely *at one* with this principle that he deduces instantly from it a stirring symphony in its entirety. This is inspiration.

The mystic touches the raw materials of creation. He does not create from secondary by-products—from theories already formulated, taught, used, and reworked—but from the original principle itself. *The mystic works with that which precedes effects; whereas the psychic works with effects.*

This is not to belittle the powers of the psychic. The student of higher sense perception who develops the ability to read effects has a valuable tool to command for self-guidance and right action. The psychic's ability to perceive effects—effects that have been experienced or are in the process of being experienced—gives him a chance to act with greater wisdom. Remember the young wife on the Nevada desert? Perceiving psychically that her husband was wandering lost in the night, she acted on this inner knowledge and saved his life. Negative events in the making may be averted through the use of HSP.

The psychic perception of effects in the process of forming is not mysterious. It is akin to what happens when a farmer sows a field of seed corn. Although he may have planted the seeds only yesterday, a field of mature corn is there today at the latent level. Someone who saw him plant the field could say, very knowingly, "A field of corn is growing here." There is no objective evidence, but the sub-surface evidence is present in the planted seed.

Events in the making are like that field of corn in the making. The effect is already present on the sub-surface or subconscious level and will manifest, barring a change in conditions. A change in weather conditions may alter the fate of the field of corn. A change—in the form of a lamp in the window—altered the fate of the husband on the Nevada desert.

How to work at the Upper Psychic Level

Jim saw immediately the difference between the lower psychic and the upper psychic level.

"What I like about the Science of Higher Sense Perception," Jim declared, "is that rather than working with techniques which permit the subconscious to assume a dominant role with little conscious direction, you emphasize keeping conscious control and simply directing the subconscious to open up new areas of power."

"Yes," I answered. "This develops *expanded* or *higher* facets of conscious-mind power, yet assures objective control of that power."

"I have wondered, though," Jim said, "whether there is some way to be certain I am working on the upper psychic level."

"Yes, of course there is. Before practicing any of the HSP training techniques, stop and consciously tell your inner mind what you want. Tell it to act discriminately. Command it to operate on the higher, pure-wisdom level. It is amenable to your suggestion and will obey your direction."

Here is a programming command similar to the one I gave Jim to use. It helped him eliminate his apprehension about HSP powers and gave him confidence that any results he demonstrated came from the higher psychic level. You, too, will wish to use it to cultivate psychic powers that tap the reliable, higher HSP levels.

Ψ   Psi-Programming Pointer
AS A PERMANENT COMMAND, I NOW DIRECT THAT *EXPANDED* CONSCIOUS POWERS WILL RESULT FROM MY PSYCHIC DEVELOPMENT—POWERS THAT TAP *HIGHER*, CONSTRUCTIVE AND RELIABLE LEVELS ONLY.

The nature of mystical experience

In this chapter, a definition of the psychic and the mystic are given to show you the difference between the levels on which HSP phenomena take place.

The psychic works with effects and effects-in-formation. The mystic works with that which precedes effects. The psychic is one who can become aware of things that are and soon will be. The mystic is one who can become aware of the principles that cause things to be. He becomes so completely *at one* with principle that sometimes the universe seems to speak or to sing to him. Such was the case with Roland B.

"This thing happened .to me over three years ago," Roland confided to me, "and I have been searching for a repeat of it ever since. This is what has brought me to the Science of Higher Sense Perception, for with your techniques, I feel that I can cultivate the mystic sense of oneness I experienced that day."

Roland then related his story, telling me of the afternoon when, finding some free time on his hands, he had driven into the mountains. He had taken along a book, thinking that he might stop somewhere and read. He parked the car in a quiet spot and went for a walk through the serene forest. He had turned his steps back when a certain rock seemed inviting, and he sat down to enjoy the columbine and other wild flowers.

"Suddenly," Roland said, "an experience occurred that changed my whole life. I've never felt despondent or frightened or lonely since. That day the universe became completely friendly."

He paused, as if uncertain as to how to go on. Groping for a way to explain to me an event that had been so extremely personal to him, he added, "I was in something of a meditative mood."

Then Roland looked straight at me and stated, "The flowers were singing! There seemed to be music everywhere."

"You're sure, of course, that you had not fallen asleep," I said. "It wasn't a dream?"

"No! I have never been so conscious in all my life before." Roland exclaimed. "I was not only awake, but I was keenly *conscious.* The feeling was not alone a heightened sense of beauty, although things did take on an added luster, but it was a feeling that took possession of me. For the first time in my life, I *knew* the meaning of oneness and I *knew* the meaning of love."

He paused and explained, "I have tried to describe this with words before, but words are so inadequate. When I speak of *knowing* love, I do not mean an experience—I *was* love, as though it were a tangible thing."

"You were both the lover and the beloved," I prompted.

My friend nodded. "That," he said, "is what I mean by oneness."

It is this sense of oneness that characterizes a mystical experience. Roland's feeling of oneness and the realization of love and kinship which springs from that feeling is what the mystics of the ages have described. Although this was a spontaneous experience for Roland—one that perhaps could not be duplicated exactly—it is possible to repeat something similar through the technique of total meditation.

In his reverie (his *meditative mood*) Roland had reached that point in consciousness where the oneness of the universe sang to him. In my serene and meditative mood in the desert hills near Phoenix, the oneness of the universe appeared to me as a symphony of expanded colors.

Beauty is in the eye of the beholder

There are various levels at which mystic and near-mystic

experiences take place. At the lower mystic level (the near-mystic) each perceiver may see quite differently, due to the filter of conditioning. Consciously and subconsciously, the individual has been conditioned to different values, outlooks, pursuits, interests, and concepts of truth and beauty. Indeed, beauty *is* in the eye of the beholder! Hence, at the near-mystic level, each beholder sees through the filter of his own consciousness, and although he honestly reports what he sees, it is subject to his own slanted interpretation.

Arthur J. Deikman, in his thesis on *experimental meditation*, explains the phenomenon of the near-mystic in these words:

> The form and content of the mystic experience is usually congruent with the mystic's cultural and religious background; to put it simply, the Yogin will have a Nirvana experience, while a Roman Catholic will report communion with Christ. Such an hypothesis of demand characteristics, however, is not consistent with the fact that the highest mystic experiences are similar in basic content despite wide differences in cultural backgrounds and expectations. These similarities are: (a) the feeling of incommunicability; (b) transcendence of sense modalities; (c) absence of specific content such as images and ideas; and (d) feeling of unity with the Ultimate.
>
> Lower forms of mystic experience do embody specific content related to each student's belief.[3]

Deikman's explanation clearly delineates the difference between the two types of mystic experience defined in the Science of Higher Sense Perception as the *lower mystic level* where impressions are received through the filtering instrument of personal culture, interest, and expectation, and the *higher mystic level* where impressions transcend personal conditioning. At the higher level, all mystics have given identical reports of a sense of oneness that is devoid of specific content but is replete with an awareness of love.

How to use the message of the mystics

One central fact stands out in the teachings of the mystics: You must change the way you view the world, if the world is to become different. It is *as* you see it!

---

[3]Deikman, Arthur J., "Experimental Meditation," *Altered States of Consciousness.* New York: John Wiley & Sons, Inc., 1969, p. 215.

What is in the eye of the beholder? How does the majority of mankind see the world? For ages, man has viewed life as a vale of tears. In his eye, it is a place of toil and trouble. He has viewed other nations as warlike and has treated his neighbor as an antagonist. He has approached strangers with suspicion and distrust because of a different language, a different culture, or a different complexion.

But the mystic has said, "Love your neighbor as yourself." Love him not as some one *like* yourself, but *as* yourself. This does not mean that you are to renounce yourself, downgrade yourself, or belittle yourself in order to exalt your neighbor. It does mean that you must respect yourself and find a self within worthy of love. Then, you can love your neighbor *as* yourself.

What will happen as more and more people change the way they behold the world? As each one rises in consciousness and sees the world rightly, a transformation will take place—not in the thing viewed, but in his view. He will begin to see the world as it has always been at the higher level of consciousness.

A higher sense perception will help man to view a world of truth and beauty that has always existed at the superconscious level. He will see the earth at last as a place of peace, harmony, and infinite richness. "Neither shall there be mourning nor crying nor pain anymore, for the former things have passed away."

At the higher mystic level, there is no feeling of separation or loneliness. Rather, there is a sense of oneness that unites mankind in a realization of love and kinship.

This is what the mystics have seen. Will you not join in this vision?

PSI-SENSITIVITY TRAINING TECHNIQUE NO. 6

SENSING A KINSHIP WITH ALL LIFE

You are seated in your favorite chair. After familiarizing yourself with this technique so you can repeat it step by step, close your eyes.

Begin by relaxing the body—this you do by first tensing the various muscles and then letting go. Start with the feet, go on to the leg muscles, the thigh, stomach, chest, and shoulder muscles.

Breathe deeply four times, holding the air for a count of four. Then exhale slowly, expelling the last residue of air before taking the next breath. As you exhale, expel every remnant of emotional and mental tension. Now, with your hands lying gently in your lap and your feet firmly placed upon the floor, let your body drift out of your consciousness.

You are aware only of your awareness. You are mind—pure mind—and there is no place you cannot go. You let yourself rise gently upward in your imagination. You drift like a balloon out the window and rise higher and higher.

It is a warm, inviting day. A gentle breeze caresses your brow. You are above the earth now, looking down upon a beautiful meadow. Although you keep rising in the air, there is no loss of the intimacy of your view. You notice in detail the delicate coloring of the meadow flowers and the trees whose leaves are dancing in the soft breeze.

On and on you seemingly rise. Your vision becomes more expansive. You see that the meadow is but one square in a patchwork quilt of fields, orchards, and pastures. As you float up and up, your vision continues to unfold. Now your view encompasses a grand sweep from the Rocky Mountains to the Alleghenies.

Still your vision grows, and gradually you see from ocean to ocean. In both directions at once, you cross the oceans and see the continent of Europe and Asia. Ceaselessly, your view embraces more and more until you behold the whole world as a globe

You feel yourself to be one with what mankind has experienced down through the eons. You are one with the thoughts of all inventors, with the wisdom of every philosopher, with the creative ideas of all thinkers, composers, and writers throughout history. You share in the psychic record of the ages. There is nothing that is inaccessible to you. But, you may lay claim to more than the psychic record of what *has been* or *now is;* you may tap the potential of all that *is to be.* Yours is more than the culmination of time in its unfoldment as form. Yours is formless time in its eternal nowness of being. You are on your way to the mystic level.

In your expanded awareness, you know yourself to be one with the whole world, with all people, with all expressions of life, with the verdant grasslands, the depthless seas, the rolling hills, and the towering mountains. As you behold all this, you mentally stretch out your arms and let them encircle the globe. You draw the world close to your breast, as a loving parent would embrace a child. In your heart you feel an overwhelming sense of love and kinship—a sense of love that radiates from your encircling arms and tells the world that it is loved, it is cared for, it is at peace.

For a few minutes in silence, you sustain the vastness of this feeling of kinship with all life. Then, slowly, you bring yourself out of the silence by counting ten, nine, eight, seven, six, five, four, three, two, one, zero, and affirm:

And so it is!

HSP SUMMARY CAPSULES

THE REAL THINGS OF LIFE

The real things of life are invisible. Unseen are the ideas behind all inventions. Invisible are the concepts of the mathematician, the composer, and the philosopher. These unseen and invisible realities never cease to be. They become a part of the vast psychic sea of subjectivity that you may tap for knowledge and guidance. Here is found a record of all that *has been* or *now is*. It can be revealed to you through the use of HSP techniques.

PSYCHIC CURRENTS OF MIND

The subjective psychic atmosphere in which man lives is not unlike the air in which the bird flies. Adverse winds may buffet him to and fro, or he may choose to glide along effortlessly on a warm up-current. You, too, may choose the psychic currents of thought you want to follow. Close to the earth are the vagrant winds of mass fears and woes. Above this is a stratum that is free from negative pollution. Stretch upward in consciousness to the pure currents of creative power!

AUTOMATIC vs. INSPIRATIONAL WRITING

To practice automatic writing, automatic speaking, or other forms of automatism is to let the psychic level express its content, independent of conscious volition. To practice *insprirational* writing is to tap the higher level of the superconscious through intuition. Inspirational writing springs from pure principle and is free from possible distortion caused by cross currents of psychic thought.

LEVELS OF PSYCHIC AND MYSTIC PERCEPTION

Just beyond the threshold of consciousness is the subjective storehouse of memory. In its collective aspect, it is the psychic record of mass living. You can tune into various compartments of this psychic powerhouse of mind, seeing images of present events, perceiving previous experiences of mankind, etc. However, beyond the psychic stratum is the superconscious level of pure mind; this is the level of the mystic

CONSCIOUS ASCENT TO MYSTIC HEIGHTS

At the central core of your being are the mystic heights where you will find the parent Cause of you. However, your ascent into those heights must come about as a conscious act of the self. Your role is one of conscious awakening. The self of you that *knows* must make the ascent. You are both the self that knows and the Self that is to be known. You are both the climber and the mountain to be climbed.

7

How to Use Directed-Dream Power for Success

It was coffee-break time in the clerical department at the bank. Clara and Louise were among the employees who were chatting together. Clara was telling about the accident in which her husband had just been involved. She related with vivid detail how the driver of the other car, a girl, had been injured. "Thank goodness it didn't turn out to be serious, though," Clara confided. "It was only a cut on the forehead and didn't require hospitalization. My husband, Clarence, wasn't hurt at all."

Louise listened as Clara chatted on about the unpleasant experience, the cost of repairs, and the inconvenience of Clarence being without a car.

A few nights later, Louise had a dream in which she saw Clara's husband in an automobile wreck. A girl was killed in the accident. Unaccountably, Louise's own family members were involved in the dream, and the accident plunged them into deep, unexplainable grief.

Next day at the bank, Louise told Clara of the dream and the dominant tone of grief that was its theme. "My whole family was in a deep state of shock; the accident turned us upside down!" Louise, troubled by the dream, continued, "Why do you suppose I dreamed of your husband, Clara?"

The two women talked it over and decided that Louise's subconscious mind—in the sleep state—had simply dramatized the incident Clara had told at coffee break. After all, Louise didn't even know Clarence except by name, and he was a complete stranger to her family. There seemed to be no point to the dream.

About three days after her dream, however, Louise's only grandson, whom she loved dearly, was killed in a car accident. She and her whole family were grieved by the news. Their lives were turned upside down. Curiously, this feeling of deep grief had been the dominant theme of Louise's dream.

Precognition in the dream state

The first conclusion that Clara and Louise had made about her dream—that the subconscious in the sleep state had simply dramatized facts she had heard at the bank—was inadequate in view of events that had now come to light.

Louise dreamed of a death. There was a death. Louise dreamed of grief into which her family was plunged. There was such grief. Clara's account of Clarence's accident became the symbolic vehicle for the precognitive impression that Louise experienced in the dream state.

The accident she had heard about during coffee break was utilized by her subconscious mind as a focal point around which to construct, symbolically, the message of her grandson's impending tragedy. There was a strong tie of love joining Louise and her grandson that formed a bond of psychic rapport between them. By the natural operation of HSP, the forthcoming accident was revealed to Louise through symbology—the language of dreams.

Although HSP phenomena such as precognition, metavision, and metaudition occur more frequently in the waking state, nothing precludes them from manifesting in the dream state. In the latter state, however, their meaning is often obscured, for it is the very nature of the dream process to dramatize a message—to veil it beneath a symbolic presentation. This is what had happened in Louise's precognitive dream.

How to utilize the HSP in your dreams

The potentialities of man's mind in the dream state must not be underrated. Not only may instances of precognition, clairvoyance, and retrocognition occur in a dream, but also intuition, guidance, creative inspiration, and artistic insight. It is a fallacy to assume that the creative, imaginative ability of the mind that functions during the waking state can be divorced from the sleep state.

It is the purpose of this chapter to make you aware of the potentialities of the sleep state so you can learn to use directed-dream power for success in all your affairs. Here is a mental area that is virtually unexplored! And it does not make sense to ignore it, for the sleep state represents almost a third of your life.

For example, if you live to be 70 years of age and you dream several dreams per night (it has been found through scientific dream monitoring that four to six dreams are normal), you will have in excess of 127,750 dreams! If there is a possibility of finding meaningful content in even *one percent* of your dreams, that possibility should not be ignored. The Science of Higher Sense Perception affirms that dreams can be utilized, and the techniques for doing so are presented in this chapter.

Pause and consider the significance of the sleep state in which you spend an excess of 23 years by the time you are 70 years of age. I want you to take advantage of these 23 years of sleeping, for their scientific utilization can make the other 47 years more creative and self-fulfilling.

You, the dreamer, awake or asleep

Awake or asleep, man is a dreamer. It might be said that the world in which he lives is a world of dreams fulfilled. The mighty bridges spanning bays and rivers, the skyscrapers, the satellites spinning through space, inventions too numerous to mention, symphonies, folk songs, poems, inspiring literature, and great art, all bespeak man's ability to dream. These are the products of a creative imaging faculty of the mind that constitutes one of the supreme mysteries of life.

This faculty displays a latitude that is seemingly unconfined. How far can this faculty take you—awake or asleep? What are the limits to this power? Without stretching the truth too far, it can be affirmed that *what the mind can conceive and believe, it can achieve!*

The imaging faculty that has been used consciously by inventors, composers, engineers, poets, statesmen, architects, and artists to construct the works of man is the same visualizing power that is at work in the dream state. It is not a different power but the same creative activity that is operating in your life whether you are awake or asleep. In fact, much of the progress of man is the result of the creative functioning of the power of imagination in the dream state.

Inestimable are the gifts to our world that have come forth through the dream process in terms of poetry, art, invention, music, and new insights in all areas. Even where insight appears to be the result of a conscious process of thought, the idea may have been conceived *first* in a dream. As Manly Palmer Hall, in *Studies in Dream Symbolism,* has said:

> A vast amount of knowledge that we now consciously hold came to us first as a result of sleep phenomena. I think if we removed from the history of knowledge all forms of scientific, philosophic, religious, cultural, artistic, esthetic, or even trade skills, that had first been revealed by dreams, we would still be in a rather primitive condition.[1]

Many famous writers credit expanded levels of mind and the dream state for their highest literary achievements—writers such as Robert Louis Stevenson who spoke of "the little people who manage man's internal theater", William Blake whose psychic sensitivity was almost compulsive in its nature, and Samuel Taylor Coleridge who produced the dramatized imagery of Kubla Khan.

Many other renowned people have found through dreams answers to mathematical problems, problems of chemistry, mechanics, and engineering. It is said that the idea of using insulin in the treatment of diabetes came to medical researcher, F. G. Banting, in a dream. Kekule von Stradonitz dreamed of the formula for the chemical, benzol. Italian composer, Tartini, wrote some of his sonatas after having heard them played by an imaginary performer in his dreams. Elias Howe, puzzling over a needle that would make the invention of a mechanical sewing machine possible, dreamed of being attacked with spears that had holes in the tips.

The list goes on and on. Indeed, it is doubtful whether any creative person of note can be left off the list of those who have

---

[1] Hall, Manly Palmer, *Studies in Dream Symbolism.* Los Angeles: The Philosophical Research Society, Inc., 1965, p. 3.

drawn upon the higher levels of mind either while dreaming, in a meditative state, or in a state of reverie.

A lot of gravel in panning a little gold

Are all dreams of great significance? Is it important to analyze every one? Will there be an element of inspiration, guidance, or insight in each dream? Let's look at it this way. In the early days of the West when a few golden flecks were discovered in a stream, often tons of gravel were panned in extracting a handful of gold nuggets. The same is true in regard to dreams. The Science of Higher Sense Perception does not purport that all dreams have a deep esoteric (hidden) significance or inspire the dreamer to create great music, art, or literature. In the first place, all dreams do not come from the same level. Most of your dreams are physical, environmental, and surface-mental. Many others are emotional, stemming from the excitements of the day. Your worries, fears, frustrations, and emotions create great mounds of gravel in the dream process.

But in-depth analyses of dreams that have been described to me by members of my dream-lab classes reveal some real golden nuggets hidden in the gravel of the sleep state—nuggets of guidance, protection, inspiration, and insight into the deeper meaning of life. What this gold has been worth to these class members in terms of self-understanding cannot be estimated.

It would be a fallacy to assume because many dreams are of a physical, environmental, and emotional nature—caused by easily understood pressures and discomforts—that *all* dreams are of a physio-emotional nature. It would be equally erroneous to assume the opposite and state that *all* dreams have some deep psychic import. The rationale of the Science of Higher Sense Perception is that there may be only three ounces of gold in a ton of dream gravel, yet these ounces are exceedingly valuable.

The corridor of your dream-consciousness

To say that you are conscious when awake and unconscious when asleep is inaccurate. I cannot conceive of *consciousness* being *unconscious.* However, I can conceive of *varying degrees or dimensions of consciousness.* Therefore, let us consider that the dream state of consciousness is a corridor along which you pass from *objective* awareness to inner, *subjective* forms of awareness.

Think of that corridor as stretching inward and upward in a series of gentle steps. At the lower end is a curtain that separates the sleeper from the waking state. At the far, upper reaches are the mystic heights that few dreamers touch. In between are roughly six levels of subjective consciousness from which dreams may arise. These are categorized in the Science of Higher Sense Perception as:

1. The Physio-environmental Level
2. The Emotional Level
3. The Surface-mental Level
4. The Lower Psychic Level (inner-mental)
5. The Upper Psychic Level (expanded-mental)
6. The Mystic Level (ascendant-mental)

For convenience in discussing these six levels, imagine that each one consists of five steps along the corridor of dreams, a total of thirty steps in all, (as depicted in Fig. 7-1.) Consider, too, that there are no actual boundaries to each level, and the dreamer may begin on the Higher Psychic Level (perhaps with elements of clairvoyance) and end on the Environmental Level as an alarm clock goes off waking the dreamer who imagines that the phone has rung.

1. THE PHYSIO-ENVIRONMENTAL LEVEL

In the phenomenon of sleep, when the cortex is sufficiently inhibited, the curtain at the lower end of the corridor is drawn shut upon outer stimuli connected with seeing, hearing, feeling, tasting, and smelling. Outer environmental factors cease to impinge upon those areas of the brain connected with sensory excitations. Then, interior stimuli begin to take over. The dreamer starts to move up the corridor of dream-consciousness.

Consider that the first five steps constitute the level on which dreams take place which are triggered by physical and environmental conditions. Objective discomforts, distractions, and crises may occur and disturb the curtain. When this happens, the dreamer may have fitful, nightmarish slumber. Or, he may have dreams that pull him back to the waking state and alert him to

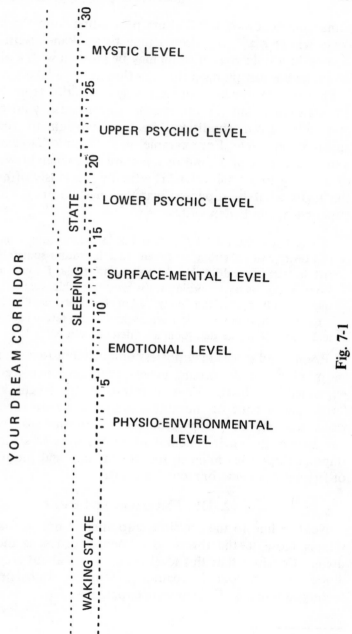

Fig. 7-1

some emergency. If the feet are protruding from the covers on a frigid winter night, the sleeper may be awakened with a dream of wading in a cold stream or he may be aroused with a nightmare in which he has just plunged through thin ice on a lake.

Physio-environmental dreams may also arise from bodily conditions such as indigestion, muscular aches, stuffy nose, etc. They may arise from conditions in the environment that are not apparent or visible. For example, in *A Study of Dreams,* Frederik van Eeden tells of a time on a lecture tour when he was the guest of a family in a small town. The family graciously offered him for the night what he supposed was the guest room. Of his resulting experience, van Eeden writes:

> I had a night full of the most horrid dreams, one long confused nightmare, with a strong sentiment that it "meant something." Yet I felt in perfect health, cheerful and comfortable. I could not refrain from saying the next morning at the breakfast table what an unpleasant night I had had. Then the family told me that I had slept in the room of a daughter who was now in a sanatorium with a severe nervous disease, and who used to call that room her "den of torture."[2]

Rooms and places may possess unique vibrations that reflect the harmonious or discordant events that have occurred there. As explained in Chapter Four in regard to the Englishwoman who "saw" the avenue of megaliths, individuals may tune into vibrations that are in the psychic record. In the case of Professor van Eeden, the environmental vibrations were so strong that they impinged upon his mind in the dream state and produced a night of fitful physio-environmental dreams.

2. THE EMOTIONAL LEVEL

·Next in line to the physio-environmental dream that keeps the sleeper close to the threshold of consciousness is the emotional dream. Consider that this level occurs from about steps six to ten along the corridor of dream-consciousness. Here the dreamer's feelings dominate his sleep-state experience.

---

[2]van Eeden, Frederik, "A Study of Dreams", *Altered States of Consciousness.* New York: John Wiley & Sons, Inc., 1969, p. 148.

Hurts, insults, indignation, resentment, or the opposite—delight, love, excitement, and joy—may determine the dream content at the Emotional Level. The feelings that motivate such dreams may arise from the current day or they may stretch back to childhood.

For example, lack of love as a child is frequently symbolized in dreams. The dreamer may see himself facing great odds completely alone. He may be struggling alone through a marshland. He may dream of being tossed on the open sea in a lifeboat without another person in sight. As his lifeboat capsizes, the scene may shift to the old swimming hole and to his near-drowning as a child. He may dream of trying to reach a smiling lady with outstretched arms, only to see her recede farther and farther away.

At the Emotional Level may be placed the wish-fulfillment dreams categorized by Freud. The emotional tensions created by moral inhibitions often find fulfillment in dream expression. Society is based upon certain limitations to the individual's freedom, and necessarily so! One person's freedom must end where the other fellow's nose begins. Tendencies of a sexual extreme must be held in check. Hatred and personal vengeance must be inhibited. Desires that are covetous, unwise, and abnormally self-centered must be re-directed.

In dreams, fortunately, emotions can express harmlessly. Many dreams are a form of wish-fulfillment. When this is so, they afford the dreamer a measure of release from pent-up emotions. Other dreams are a form of guidance, symbolically telling the dreamer how he can solve his emotional problems. Such was true of a dream Steve M. had repeatedly.

How a dream solved an emotional problem

Steve, a member of a class I gave on dream interpretation, had a recurring dream that puzzled him. He agreed to submit it for analysis during a dream-lab session.

"It always begins with a beautiful day," Steve explained. "The sun is shining and I can feel a gentle breeze across my brow. Suddenly, I find myself in a zoo. I am alone. No one else is there. I am entering a huge red building with a long hall of arches. On either side of the hall are animals in cages—two of each specie. Underfoot are tropical plants and giant snakes."

"These animals are not of ordinary size; they're many times their normal proportion. As I watch, they become restless, and two elephants break loose and stampede out of the hall. Suddenly, two giant lions seem to flow out of a cage filled with water. With this, I find myself climbing the arches of the building. I inch up higher and higher. Finally at the top of an arch, I look down and the animals are small. From that great height, I feel very safe and very light."

Steve was a big man, the kind you would think could lick his weight in wild cats. He did not seem like one who would run away from anything, but he had been dodging his emotions for years. He was sensitive and felt things keenly. The force of his emotions frightened him, and he had never dared let them show. This was symbolized in his dream.

"Steve," I said, "look at your dream this way. The animals represent your emotions, emotions that you are afraid have become oversize. The water in dream symbolism is the psychic sea, the sea of accumulated past experiences. In climbing the arch of the building, you reduce your emotions to their normal size. By getting above the situation, you're safe—you're in control."

"It's true," Steve confided. "For years I *have* been trying to repress my emotions and keep them under control."

"But repression isn't a real solution. Your dream is telling you to get *above* your emotions, and they'll take on a normal size. Like the ferocious lions that were reduced in size and in their power to hurt, emotions—no matter how unruly—can be reduced as a threat to happiness. Not by repression, but by sublimation!

"Sublimating emotional force means using it for creative purposes. It means putting it in right perspective. It means climbing to a higher level of the Self where you are director of (not directed by) your emotions."

Steve was excited about the interpretation. He saw at once what his dream had been trying to tell him, and he was determined not to run away from his emotions again. He decided to face them and direct them deliberately toward creative pursuits.

It was perhaps a month after the end of the course that I saw Steve again. He looked happy and very relaxed. I asked him about his dream. "Has it ever come back?" Steve smiled and shook his head NO.

Directed-Dream Power calls for emotional control

Steve had taken a step essential to the use of directed-dream power. He had eliminated a recurring dream by wiping out its emotional cause. Also, he had discovered how meaningful the content of a dream is in helping him understand himself.

If you are to utilize dream-power creatively as explained as this chapter unfolds, you must eliminate needless emotional dreams. Learn to become director of your emotions by giving them lofty outlets. Climb to a higher level of the Self, as Steve did, where emotional force will express as creative energy, inspirational vigor, and constructive enthusiasm.

Program your mind and emotions with the following command to the subconscious:

Ψ   Psi-Programming Pointer

FROM A LOFTY VANTAGE POINT, I DIRECT THE DYNAMIC FORCE OF MY EMOTIONS. THIS FORCE FLOWS UNOBSTRUCTEDLY INTO CREATIVE PURSUITS, BRINGING ME HAPPINESS AND SUCCESS.

---

3. THE SURFACE-MENTAL LEVEL

The dream state frequently becomes a continuation of the intellectual challenges and mental concerns with which the individual's waking hours are filled. Dreams of this nature may be classified as surface-mental dreams. They are the symbolic continuation of the lines-of-thought that occupy the dreamer's conscious state. Consider that these dreams occur between steps eleven and fifteen along the corridor of subjective consciousness.

A certain mental theme may dominate an individual's waking line-of-thought. If so, that theme may invade his dream-world in various forms or may repeat as the same recurring dream. This is especially true of mental or philosophical quandaries that go unresolved.

Lester T., another member of my dream course, had a recurring dream that illustrates how intellectual concerns may result in a surface-mental dream.

How a dream indicates surface-mental concerns

Three or four times a year Lester's dream repeated itself. It invariably started at the same point. "In my dream," Lester said, "I am always crawling through a large machine. There are dozens of wheels turning and rotating at various speeds. Some wheels are the size of small gears that one might find in a watch: some are huge wheels as big as a building! I find myself laboriously trying to wind my way through them, and at times I am in danger of being crushed!"

The dream was symbolic, of course. It seemed to say that Lester was going round and round a problem—questioning, agonizing, wondering but never coming to a decision.

What was Lester's problem, the one that kept him in a torment of indecision? Well, for years Lester had referred to himself as an atheist. However, an atheist is one who stoutly disbelieves and is certain about his disbelief. Lester was not *all* that certain. Philosophical and theological questions plagued him. He would look first to one answer and then to another, never able to resolve his doubts. Lester was—more accurately—an agnostic, a questioner.

In his dream, the wheels that kept turning were the questions that kept grinding through his head. Crawling through the gears symbolized his attempt to find his way among the conflicting philosophical and theological theories he questioned. I suggested that the dream probably would not come to a halt until he stopped going round and round and came to a conclusion.

At first, Lester was a little miffed by my interpretation of his dream. In effect, I had told him that he was confused, and he felt I was not too kind. However, he quickly saw that truth was going to help him more than kindness. "I guess," he said, "for my own peace of mind I'll have to take some solid stand. If that stand later proves unsatisfactory, I can always change it."

A recurring dream such as Steve's or Lester's is symbolic feedback from the subconscious. If you have a recurring dream, it may point up areas that need your conscious analysis and action. It may show you a facet of your life where confusion, inadequacy, indecision, annoyance, or uncertainty exist.

Dreams are one way that the Real Self can speak to you. In a sense that Self is saying, "Get with it! Wake up and recognize the problems that are begging for solution. Stop postponing decisions you need to make!"

Learn to heed the subconscious feedback from the interior Self that comes during the dream state and utilize it. This is making directed-dream power work for you!

4. THE LOWER PSYCHIC LEVEL

The dream state, as explained in Fig. 7-1, is like a corridor leading from objective awareness upward or inward to subjective levels of consciousness. At the first level, physio-environmental forces from the objective world around a sleeper may influence his dreams. At the second level, excitement or distress from the day may contribute to emotionally motivated dreams. At the third level, a sleeper's current mental preoccupations may carry over into symbolic dream experiences.

At the fourth level, which may be considered as steps sixteen to twenty, dreams arise from stimuli that are more interior. They belong to the inner-mental or deep-memory level. Man's mind is like a microfilm library, and lining his mental shelves are reel after reel of pictures he has taken. This is his *personal psychic record.* Here in deep storage are all the impressions that go toward making up his self-image, his image of his fellowman, and his image of the scheme of things. All that he has experienced is filed away in these deep recesses of subjective mind.

This is the Lower Psychic Level, and dreams that arise from it may involve incidents of last month, last year, or last lifetime. Whatever is indelibly etched on the personal psychic record is subject to review in the dream state.

In Chapter 10 you will find an account of my own experience with psychic-record dreaming—a phenomenon that involves deep-memory perception. The experience of a former life, stored away in an individual's personal psychic record, may become the content of a dream.

5. THE HIGHER PSYCHIC LEVEL

The next area along the corridor of dream-consciousness is designated in Fig. 7-1 as the Higher Psychic Level. It corresponds to the level of expanded mental powers in the waking state where man may experience telepathy, precognition, retrocognition, metavision (clairvoyance), metaudition, etc.

Here, in the dream state, the sleeper may experience instances of guidance, prophecy, and premonition in symbolic form. Louise's precognitive dream of the death of her favorite grandson in a car accident belongs to this level.

History is replete with dreams that belong to this category. Ancient kings made a practice of keeping soothsayers to advise them on the interpretation of prophetic dreams. Among the most renowned advisors was Joseph, who served the Pharaoh of Egypt brilliantly in this capacity.

Joseph's talents first came to the attention of the Pharaoh after he had a particularly vivid and disturbing dream. After searching the length of the land for someone who could interpret it, Joseph, a prisoner in the Pharaoh's own dungeon, was recommended to him. This is what he related to Joseph:

> In my dream I was standing on the bank of the Nile; up came seven cows, plump and sleek, and they grazed in the reed-grass. After them seven other cows came up, starved and very ugly and lean—I never saw such poor cows in all the land of Egypt. The lean and ugly cows ate up the first seven plump cows . . . then I woke up. Next I saw in a dream seven full ripe ears sprouting on a single stalk. Seven ears sprang up after them, withered, thin, and blasted by the east wind, and the thin ears swallowed up the seven ripe ears! (Genesis 41:14-24)

Upon hearing the dream, Joseph told the Pharaoh that the seven good cows were seven good years and the seven lean cows were seven years of famine. The second dream said exactly the same thing with different symbols—the seven ripe ears represented seven lush years; the seven thin ears symbolized seven draught years.

Joseph then suggested that the king appoint a shrewd, intelligent man to control the land during the seven years of abundance, laying aside a fifth of the harvest each year to provide for the years of famine. This the Pharaoh did, appointing Joseph himself as the food-controller, and Egypt survived during the lean and ugly years of famine.

Joseph possessed an uncanny talent for sifting significant dreams—those with golden nuggets of guidance and insight—from the insignificant "gravel" of ordinary dreams.

A case of HSP guidance through directed-dream power

"So what," you may say. "I am not a Joseph." No, but you may be a Kent.

Kent had worked most of his life for others. He loved good foods and was an excellent chef. His services were always in demand, but he wanted to try his skill in a restaurant of his own.

Kent heard of an opportunity to buy a place that he felt needed only his culinary ability to prosper. To reach the deal financially, however, he needed more money than he had saved. His credit rating was good, so he was not worried about *borrowing enough—* but he was concerned about *making enough* to pay back the loan Could he succeed?

Kent considered me both a counselor and a friend, and he sought me out for advice. "I've never worked for myself before. Do you think I am kidding myself? Do you think I can swing it?"

I told him that it was much more important what he thought than what I thought. "Kent, by using your own HSP powers, you can let guidance come through. First, of course, you must analyze the proposition *consciously* to see if it is a smart move to take. But then, before your final decision, feed a guidance command into the *subconscious.* Let the higher, extended power of your own mind guide you in your final choice. Your inner mind can perceive ramifications and consequences that the limited conscious mind just isn't capable of!"

Kent had been a member of one of my dream classes and was interested in trying out directed-dream power to help him with his final decision.

How to use dreams for YES or NO answers

I reminded Kent that as he slipped off to sleep he could phrase a command for guidance in YES or NO terms. "For a YES or *go ahead* answer, you direct that you'll dream of something green. For a NO or *stop* answer, you direct that you'll dream of something red."

"A more general approach to guidance," I continued, "is to look for answers in dream situations. You may wish simply to direct that the RIGHT SOLUTION be made clear to you some-place in the content of your dream."

This approach appealed to Kent, and he decided to try it. For several nights he followed detailed training similar to the HSP Sensitivity Training Technique given at the end of this chapter. He kept a pad and pencil by his bed, as I suggested, and recorded his dreams as soon as he awoke.

A few days later, Kent had this dream to relate to me—one that was to both of us a clear case of interior guidance:

"In my dream, I was visiting a friend. His face was not clear and it was no one I could name, but he was unmistakably a wise and valued friend.

"I was explaining my idea of buying this restaurant to him. My friend listened and then encouraged me to go ahead, urging me in a kind but very insistent manner. My dream-friend told me that the move would be the most successful endeavor of my life!"

Kent felt strongly that he should go ahead. With this encouragement, he borrowed the necessary capital and bought the restaurant. Today, he has a highly successful business. His dream-friend was right!

Why not turn your dreams into a friend by using directed-dream power! To ignore your mind in the dream state is to ignore almost half of your power to think.

6. THE MYSTIC LEVEL

The highest point along the dream corridor that the sleeper may reach is the Mystic Level. Like the other levels, it is comprised of a sliding series of degrees or steps—steps that blend imperceptibly one into the other.

Consider that the steps stretch from twenty-six to thirty on the dream-consciousness scale. It is here that dreams of intuition occur. Here the mind, tapping pure principles, produces inspiration for the inventor, the artist, the researcher, the writer, and the composer whose dreams have been significant.

At the highest step along the corridor, a dream-state few ever attain, man reaches into the mystic dimensions of the real Self. Here occurs the feeling of oneness of which the mystic speaks—a feeling that may be experienced in the dream state on rare occasions of high consciousness. Here man sometimes is able to part the curtain at the upper end of the dream corridor and catch a glimpse into the mystery of the superconscious.

Applying directed-dream power for success

A new realm of potential power awaits you in the sleep phenomena of dreams. Some dreams may carry nothing more than psychic feedback from daily preoccupations. But, others may carry elements of creative inspiration. Still others may carry elements of precognition and guidance.

To utilize this new potential for wisdom, guidance, and success, start now to re-educate your attitudes toward dreams:

First, cultivate an attitude of respect for your dreams. You must feel that your dreams are rational—although that rationality is often obscure. You do not have a *rational* awake state and an *irrational* sleep state.

Don't remark, "Oh, it was only a dream," downgrading your dreams is if they have no relationship to you. They are just as much a part of your life as your waking thoughts. Respect yourself in the sleep state as you do yourself in the awake state.

Second, assume control over your dream-life. Up to now you may have felt that you had no power over the dream process, but this need not be! Cultivate the idea that you have control over your *entire* psychic life—awake *and* asleep.

You can direct the psychic forces that have spewed forth in idle and confused dreaming. You can learn to dream upon demand. You can give your dreams something constructive to do—problems to solve, answers to formulate. You are not the victim of your dreams, but their cause. And, you can be their control!

Third, use directed-dream power to learn more about yourself. In their own way, your dreams are saying something meaningful to you, and you can learn from what is being said. At the Physio-environmental Level, dreams may be saying, "Don't over-eat before going to bed." At the Emotional Level, dreams may reveal an intolerence, an impatience, a lack of forgiveness, a surly temper, etc. Listen to the feedback from your dreams and learn from it!

Fourth, use directed-dream power to solve problems. As you retire for bed, put the problem in the hopper of the subconscious for solution during the night. How do you do this? By using the HSP technique given at the end of this chapter. Know that an inner wisdom—a good friend as was the case with Kent—is ever able to guide you into making RIGHT DECISIONS. Believe that an answer will come, either by means of a dream or some revealing hunch during the day.

Fifth, use dream-therapy to uncover tensions and resentments. Have a dream-therapy session around the breakfast table each morning. Inner feelings revealed in dream content may point out areas where more love and consideration are needed in family life.

For example, a child's dreams may reveal hostilities building up on the inner plane toward brothers, sisters, or society, that if unrevealed can become a Pandora's Box of trouble. Parents could resolve many unsuspected tensions and resentments—and help their families to healthier living—by encouraging children to express their dreams in regular dream-therapy sessions.

What to do with symbology in your dreams

There are dozens of dream-symbol *dictionaries* on the market that categorically list specific definitions for specific symbols. In the Science of Higher Sense Perception, however, it has been found that the interpretation of dream symbols is a personal art that you must learn to perform for yourself.

True, there are certain archetypal symbols that seem to reappear and carry consistent meanings such as an *old woman,* an *old man,* a *dark chasm,* a *dark pool,* the *water of the psychic sea,* a *mountain,* etc. In the writings of Carl G. Jung, you can find much of value to make you familiar with these archetypal patterns. However, the final meaning of any symbol lies in your own consciousness and the experiences you have gone through.

For example, a mountain traditionally symbolizes a sense of aspiration. Hence, the person who dreams of climbing a mountain—perhaps finding a gleaming-white cathedral at the top— must be aspiring upward to the higher ground of his being. However, consider what meaning a mountain may have for a person who as a child was lost in an alpine wilderness. For him the mountain may symbolize despair.

What do you do with the symbology in your dreams? Remember that dream symbols, to a great degree, are unique to your own consciousness, and the interpretation of them is a personal art. How do you go about developing that art? Use this method:

Following the detailed instructions in the next section, write out your dream. Pay particular attention to key words and concepts. Then, ask yourself what these key features mean to you. Do not accept the literal meaning.

For example, if you dream of a relative, interpret his appearance as a representation of some state of consciousness within yourself. If you dream of your brother, don't say, "Last night I dreamed of my brother Bob." Say rather, "I dreamed of me, in which my brother Bob represents some quality or meaning for me. What does my brother mean to me? Does he represent something I admire or despise?"

In most every case, you are the dreamer dreaming about you. Your dream is a personal experience. The more you work with dreams, the greater will become your skill in the art of interpreting personal dream symbols.

The techniques of dream retrieval and interpretation

To harness the array of subjective data you encounter along the dream corridor, you must know how to capture your dreams and recall them the next morning for analysis. To retrieve your dreams, take these steps:

First, keep a pencil and notebook beside your bed to use only for the recording of dreams.

Second, strongly suggest to yourself several times before you fall asleep, *I will remember my dreams!* This is essential, especially if you are one of those people who asserts that he never dreams. The mind has been conditioned to conceal dreams by sweeping away their content upon awakening.

Third, observe yourself while dreaming. This you do by commanding, before you fall asleep, that you will be able to observe the dream process and its significance.

Fourth, write out the main features of your dreams the moment you awaken. Record key words and concepts. Make your interpretation of symbols a personal art.

Fifth, look for the lesson your dream seeks to reveal or the answer it gives to some question you posed before going to sleep. Be practical and honest in your dream interpretation. Remember, the meaning must satisfy you, the dreamer.

Sixth, persist in the practice of using your dreams for guidance. Persist in panning your dreams for the golden nuggets they may contain. Proficiency in any area of accomplishment comes from repeated practice.

Seventh, use the Psi-Sensitivity Training Technique that follows before going to sleep each night. As you meditate, direct that the meaning of your dreams will be revealed to you. Stay alert if you are using this technique in bed, and do not slip off to sleep until you have finished your mental training.

Eighth, be grateful for the avenue of wisdom and guidance you can tap through directed use of the dream-state. Gratitude for meaningful dreams is the key that unlocks their content.

PSI-SENSITIVITY TRAINING TECHNIQUE NO. 7

TAPPING DREAM POWER FOR GUIDANCE

This training technique is to be practiced just before going to sleep. Use it to tap the higher dream levels for guidance, answers to problems, insight, inspiration, and intuition.

You are lying in your bed. You release physical pressures from the body by tensing and relaxing each muscle in turn as you have done previously in other psi-training sessions. In addition, you speak to each part of the body and command it to relax, and your body responds to your word. Next, you speak to your subconscious mind and command it to listen and obey. It is the servant of the conscious mind, and it will respond to your word of authority.

With your eyes closed, you now picture before you a large blackboard. Upon the blackboard you now write mentally in large white letters the question for which you seek an answer, the guidance you wish to demonstrate, the insight you wish to attain. You phrase the matter that requires an answer in clear, concise terms. You form each white chalk-like word distinctly and deliberately.

At the same time, your lips form the words and you silently speak them with firmness and with confidence—confidence that asleep or awake expanded powers are available to you. Speak your word of command to the real Self, directing that the RIGHT SOLUTION to the matter at hand be made known to you.

When your request has been written once in mental letters upon the blackboard of mind and spoken, you erase it from your mind's eye. Then, you write it again—boldly and confidently. Speak it again, and then erase it. For the third time, write it, speak your word, and erase it—knowing in your heart that a RIGHT SOLUTION exists and that it will be made known to you.

Remembering that symbology is the language of dreams, you may wish to command that the answer to a request for guidance (or any matter that can be answered "yes" or "no") be given to you in terms of a specific symbol. For a "yes" answer, you may direct that you shall dream of something green—grass, trees—for a "no" answer, something red. In any event, give a command to the subconscious to reveal the RIGHT SOLUTION to you in symbols that are meaningful and will be comprehended immediately by you as you awake in the morning.

End your psi-training now with a feeling of absolute expectation of guidance and inspiration. You have placed your order. You have spoken your word! You have a *feeling of certainty* that results will be delivered to you—the same certainty you would have if you ordered something by mail and were awaiting its delivery. A RIGHT SOLUTION is on its way!

Lying in bed, you slip off to sleep now in the firm expectation that your higher-sense-perception powers will reveal to you, during the dream state, the answer or guidance or insight you seek. You go to sleep with a feeling of accomplishment—with the feeling that you now have the wise counsel you seek. In this feeling of accomplishment, there is no room for doubt or anxiety. There is only a calmness, an assurance and a deep realization of gratitude.

As you drift off to sleep in this feeling of expectation and gratitude, you silently affirm:

And so it is!

SUMMARY CAPSULES

AWAKE OR ASLEEP, YOU ARE A DREAMER

The creative, imaginative ability that functions during the waking state cannot be divorced from the dream state. Both awake and asleep, man is capable of conceiving creative ideas that bring progress, achievement, and release from drudgery. During the phenomenon of sleep, you may dream of the solution to a problem or perceive the idea for an invention. You may be inspired to write or compose or paint.

SYMBOLISM MUST FIT YOU, THE DREAMER

The content of a dream frequently masquerades beneath an altered mask, for symbolism is the language of dreams. The subconscious speaks in cryptic, capricious ways, and it may not re-use a symbol twice to convey the same meaning. Therefore, the interpretation of dream symbolism is a matter that must be handled by the dreamer himself. To be the right interpretation, it must fit you, the dreamer.

YOUR DREAMS ARE SUBCONSCIOUS FEEDBACK

A general interpretation of your dreams can help you understand problems confronting the mind that are begging for solution. Often, dreams are the subconscious feedback from unfulfilled desires, unresolved concerns, and unrealized aspirations. You can use this feedback to help you identify areas where work can be done to solve problems and establish peace of mind.

YOUR DREAM CORRIDOR OF SUBJECTIVITY

As the curtain of sleep closes across the threshold of consciousness, you enter a dream corridor. This corridor stretches inward and upward, leading from objective awareness to inner levels of subjectivity—the physio-environmental, the emotional, the surface-mental, the lower psychic, the upper psychic, and the mystic. During the dream experience, you are led randomly along the corridor, unless you train yourself to direct your dreams.

HOW TO USE DIRECTED-DREAM POWER

Although much of the roaming done by the mind during sleep is capricious, you can harness the subconscious and put it to work for you during the dream state. Before going to sleep, program a command into the subconscious. Direct it to work on some question you wish answered. Direct the real Self to reveal its wisdom through the symbology of your dreams. The use of directed-dream power can double your thinking time.

8

How to Overcome Any
Fear of the Astral World

The young lady seated across the table from me didn't look ill. She displayed emotional stability, and, certainly, if she had been psycho-neurotic, she could not have kept the good job she held in the accounting field. Aside from being a little underweight, she appeared to be healthy in body and mind.

But Gladys was worried about herself. She said, "I have moments when I seem to be outside my body looking at my physical form, just as I am looking at you now. Why, the other day," she exclaimed, "I was trying to meditate, when I seemed to float outside myself. I found myself up toward the ceiling looking down at my body as though I were two people."

Gladys went on to explain her anxiety about these occasional sensations of disassociation she was experiencing. They frightened her, and she feared they were a sign of mental illness. Of course, there *are* psychotic disorders and hallucinations that cause loss of contact with environment but this was not the case with Gladys. Mentally, she was self-integrated. She related well with her environment.

This young lady's out-of-the-body sensations stemmed from a higher-sense-perception capacity that every individual has because of the very nature of his being: That nature is defined as a *consciousness that has a body* rather than a body that has consciousness. Remember, consciousness is something greater than the body, and it is not confined to the body.

This thing that is greater is the *real Self.* It is the non-material *essence* that clothes itself in form for experience in the time-space world. It is the *essential core* from which the five known physical senses spring. It is the *essence* which is capable of *higher* sense perception.

For the most part, the non-material real Self functions through the body. But this does not preclude its functioning above and beyond the body. This is what happens in the kind of out-of-the-body sensations that Gladys had. In quiet, contemplative moments she spontaneously projected her consciousness above and beyond the physical vehicle of expression. Although the projection was not intentional on her part and frightened her badly, it is possible to cultivate the technique deliberately and find it pleasurable.

Some instances of projection-in-consciousness

Gladys' problem, I felt, would be solved when she understood just what happens during an out-of-the-body sensation.

First, no exterior force is responsible for the experience. Hence, there is no external influence to fear.

Second, it is a phenomenon that has been cultivated without harm by many who explore the HSP field.

Third, the individual has the power to control and direct such experiences through conscious commands to the subconscious mind. The full prerogative to induce the sensation again or to terminate any future recurrence of it lies with the individual himself.

To allay Gladys' fear that she was abnormal, I told her of a number of similar accounts reported to me by people who had sensations of viewing their bodies from above—usually from a corner of the room. Many of these sensations occur while the individual is resting and awake. Others occur on the borderland of sleep where the individual cannot be sure whether he is awake or dreaming.

Some out-of-the-body sensations are very simple, as was Gladys'. Others are very comprehensive "trips" in consciousness. An elderly gentlemen, quite scholarly and spiritual, who lived at the

Brown Palace in Denver planned his "astral trips" as definitely as the ordinary person plans a motor tour. He was known to cancel afternoon appointments in order to schedule his projections-in-consciousness to his liking. Then, he would seat himself quietly in his hotel room (with his hat on) and take an astral journey to a scene of his choice.

"But how did he come by the ability to do this?" Gladys asked. Here is the explanation that helped her understand why some people may experience such phenomenon while others do not. It will help you, too, to understand and work with your HSP potentialities.

Why are some people able—whether intentionally or unintentionally—to experience sensations beyond the physical while other people seem rigidly bound to the body?

The answer lies simply in the fact that the body dominates the attention for most people. They are slavishly identified with the physical form for they have not explored the possibility that the real Self is non-material.

But non-material the Self must be, for it is the indestructible factor that gives you continuity of personality, individuality, and memory through change after change of body. Physiologically, you have a different body today than you had a few years ago. Constantly, new cells are formed to replace the old that die. Continually, you grow new hair, new nails, new epidermis cells—and the old are gone. Energy is burned up. Enzymes and vital fluids are used up and replaced by new.

Yet, no element of your awareness is used up, gone, or lost. Why? Because the indestructible Self that creates new cells is non-material. The real Self is an enduring reality that is greater than the physical vehicle. The real Self is the changeless, eternal YOU behind all change.

Your non-material vehicle of expression

Start today to realize that you have a body, *not* that your body has you! The real Self simply projects the physical body as a material vehicle of expression. The material level is the most tangible or dense form of matter. The real Self uses the body for material experiences.

For non-material experiences, the real Self uses a less tangible body sometimes referred to as the astral body. A dictionary defines *astral* as *"a supersensible substance (a substance beyond physical senses) held to be next above the tangible world in refinement."* When your consciousness is experiencing outside the body, you may think of it as functioning through an astral body—using a non-physical body as its vehicle of expression.

The term *astral* comes from occult teachings which hold that the astral body is one of several bodies through which the Self functions on various levels of its being. The Self, on its upward journey, manifests a vehicle of expression appropriate to the level it has attained, stretching from the physical—the most dense—up to the superconscious where the intangible substance of pure idea is reached.

What is the finer substance of astral matter?

What are the components of matter—be it dense or fine? All physical matter can be reduced to molecules, and molecules to atoms, and atoms to electrons, protons, and neutrons. These infinitesimal units of matter, in turn, are simply electrical charges of energy. Hence, all matter is really energy. When it is dense, it is *visible*. When it is less dense, it is *invisible* to the normal eye.

Now, let's go one step further in the analysis of matter and postulate that those infinitesimal units of energy which make up all substance may be defined as units of mind. Thus, energy is mind! If so, *the power of mind over matter* is no mystery. Both are really composed of the same substance, but that which is higher in consciousness (the mind) has power over that which is lower or more dense (the body).

The mind does not function in the same restricted world as the physical body. It is not bound to the same material laws. To the mind, distance is no barrier, and time and space do not exist as limiting dimensions. The same is true of the astral body. It is a mental body, and distance is no barrier to it.

For example, when you think about a loved one, he *comes* to mind instantly, but that *coming* is not in terms of distance from some place. The meeting occurs in mind, not in space. When you "go" someplace by means of the astral body, distance is not a factor. The trip takes place in consciousness

An astral visit that spanned 1,000 miles

One such meeting *in consciousness* took place for a husband and wife separated by a thousand miles of Atlantic Ocean. In the *Proceedings of the Society for Psychical Research*, G. N. M. Tyrrell relates this curious account involving a rough crossing of the Atlantic Ocean. S. R. Wilmot, an American, was returning to his wife in New York. On the voyage, he shared a stateroom with a Mr. Tait. Their berths were constructed so that the top one set back farther than the lower one—thus the two were not vertically over one another. Wilmot occupied the lower berth and Tait, the top.

Tyrrell, a mathematician who pioneered *quantitative* psychical research, relates the strange event that took place one night in Wilmot's cabin:[1]

> After eight days of bad weather, Mr. Wilmot was enjoying his first night of refreshing sleep, when, as he says, "Towards morning I dreamt that I saw my wife, whom I had left in the United States, come to the door of my stateroom, clad in her night dress. At the door she seemed to discover that I was not the only occupant of the room, hesitated a little, then advanced to my side, stooped down and kissed me and after gently caressing me for a few moments, quietly withdrew.
>
> Upon waking up I was surprised to see my fellow passenger... leaning upon his elbow and looking fixedly at me. "You're a pretty fellow," he said at length, "to have a lady come and visit you in this way." I pressed for an explanation... and at length he related what he had seen while wide awake, lying in his berth. It exactly corresponded with my dream.
>
> The narrator went on to say, "On arriving home and meeting my wife, almost her first question when we were alone together was, 'Did you receive a visit from me a week ago Tuesday?' 'A visit from you?' said I. We were more than a thousand miles at sea.' 'I know it,' she replied, 'but it seemed to me that I visited you.' "
>
> "My wife then told me that on account of the severity of the weather and the reported loss of the *Africa* ... she had been extremely anxious about me. On the same night when the storm had just begun to abate, she had lain awake for a long time thinking of me, and about four o'clock in the morning it seemed to her that she went out to seek me."

---

[1]Tyrrell, G. N. M., *Science and Psychical Phenomena and Apparitions* (in one volume). New York: University Books, Inc., 1961, Vol. 2, p. 116-117.

"Crossing the wide and stormy sea, she came at length to a low, black steamship, whose side she went up and then descended into the cabin, passed through it to the stern until she came to my stateroom. 'Tell me,' she said, 'do they ever have staterooms like the one I saw where the upper berth extends further back than the under one? A man was in the upper berth looking right at me, and for a moment I was afraid to go in, but soon I went up to the side of your berth, bent down and kissed you and embraced you and then went away.' " [1]

Tyrrell, in commenting on this phenomenon says, "It may, I think, be doubted whether Mr. Wilmot's experience was, properly speaking, a dream." [2]

How experiences take place independently of the body

Is the spirit never free to roam? Is it restricted by the confines of time and space? Is the real Self body-bound and limited to physical expression? The answer of the Science of Higher Sense Perception is NO! The power of mind over matter is real. Experiences may take place in mind that are independent of the body. Meetings may occur in mind and projections of consciousness (astral travel) may be experienced because:

1. The mind is not the garment-of-flesh in which it is enclosed. The real Self is greater than its clothing, whether the clothing be the physical form or the environment that seems to hem it in.

2. The body is a physical observation tower for the real Self, the real observer. The Self, however, is not confined to this tower. It may function through the less dense observation tower of the astral form.

3. Thought is the motive power of astral travel. A person is always projecting himself before him in terms of thought. He literally goes where his thought takes him. He travels on the wings of thought.

Hence, in these three points, are factors that explain the experience of Wilmot, his wife, and Tait, his traveling companion. Mrs. Wilmot was concerned for the safety of her husband; she needed reassurance of his well being. In her anxious state of thought, she mentally went in search of her husband. Whether or not she fell into a dream state, her physical body lay in a bed in

[2]*Ibid.*, P. 117.

New York while an observing self reduced a thousand miles of ocean to nothingness and visited the bedside of her husband.

Whether or not Mr. Wilmot was dreaming of his wife, their thoughts did in some way synchronize and function on the same HSP level, a mutual level of experience shared by both. It is significant that Wilmot was relaxing well for the first time in eight nights, putting him in a receptive state of consciousness.

Tait, who believed himself awake, was also receptive and tuned into a mental program that was being broadcast at an astral level of consciousness. He, too, was functioning through his observing self on a mental level of awareness.

It is interesting to speculate, had impersonal parties been present in these two locations, what would have been reported about these three participants. Were Mr. and Mrs. Wilmot both asleep, while Tait was awake? Were all three in a sleep state? Were Tait and Mrs. Wilmot in a state more akin to meditation, while Wilmot was asleep? Regardless of their states, the experience shared by these three was real to them. They were participants in a meeting at an interior level of consciousness—an HSP level.

Double-body sensations in the dream state

When astral projection occurs in a dream state, the body is asleep but the real Self is very much awake. It *knows* the body is sleeping. It usually experiences the sensation of looking down and beholding the body resting peacefully on the bed. There may be a distinct sensation of having two bodies.

Frederik van Eeden, researcher on dreams who has categorized them into nine different types, recorded many of his own dreams over the years. Speaking of the *lucid* type, he writes of the double-body sensation he experienced:[3]

> The night of January 19, I dreamt that I was lying in the garden before the window of my study, and saw the eyes of my dog through the glass pane. I was lying on my chest and observing the dog keenly.
>
> At the same time, however, I knew with perfect certainty that I was dreaming and lying on my back in my bed. And then I resolved to wake up slowly and carefully and observe how my sensation of lying on my chest would change at the sensation of lying on my back. And so I did,

---

[3]van Eeden, Frederik, *op. cit.,* p. 151.

slowly and deliberately, and the transition—which I have since undergone many times—is most wonderful. It is like the feeling of *slipping from one body into another,* and there is distinctly a double recollection of the two bodies.

van Eeden had the distinct sensation of being outside his physical body, observing it from a second self. I feel this was an instance of astral projection while the body was in sleep state. His observing self, for the moment, was experiencing through the astral body—a less dense, less tangible form.

Astral projection is not a dream. It does occur, however, while a person is in a quiescent state. It *may* happen while an individual is resting, or sitting in quiet reverie, or sleeping, or practicing meditation. This was the case with Gladys. Her out-of-the-body sensations occurred while she was quieting herself for meditation. For the moment, her observing self functioned through the less tangible vehicle of the astral form which is freer and less restricted than the physical body.

Why did this happen to her? Basically, she was less body-bound than the average person. Gladys was an alert, inquisitive thinker who found her inner potentialities fascinating. She was just beginning to cultivate those powers through meditation, but she had not done much to direct her energies as yet. She needed to step from non-direction into direction of her HSP potentialities.

Although there was no need for Gladys to fear the out-of-the-body sensations she had told me about, there was a need to *overcome* that fear. She needed to learn that she was in control of her mind at all times. She needed to demonstrate that she was commander-in-chief of her consciousness and that no outside influence produced these phenomena. Once certain of this, she could then go on to perfect her "astral travel" if she so desired.

I gave Gladys an affirmation similar to the following Psi-Programming Pointer to use each time she sat down to rest, or to sleep, or to meditate. Its purpose was to program her subconscious mind with an edict that lodged all control with the conscious mind—control you, too, may need to overcome fear and gain self-confidence.

Gladys used the Pointer to program her subconscious mind and it worked! She commanded that she experience nothing she did not *consciously* choose to experience. She commanded that she feel no sensations she did not *consciously* wish to feel. She commanded that she retain control to begin and end all HSP phenomena at her *conscious* pleasure. She affirmed that no out-of-the-body sensations would occur unless she deliberately willed them to. Her fear disappeared! She knew, at last, that there was no force waiting to usurp her will or use her mind capriciously.

She became "the master of her fate and the captain of her soul" as anyone can who uses this Psi-Programming Pointer and HSP Sensitivity Training Technique No. 8 on psychic protection at the end of the chapter.

Ψ   Psi-Programming Pointer

MY CONSCIOUS MIND IS THE RULING, CONTROLLING, DIRECTING SIDE OF MY REAL SELF. MY SUBCONSCIOUS MIND OBEYS AND NEVER EXCEEDS THE CONSCIOUS MIND COMMANDS I GIVE IT.

Astral projection as apparitions

In a class of mine on HSP, I told them of Gladys' encounter with projection of the astral body. Some had experienced similar out-of-the-body sensations and were relieved to discover a means of control. Others had various apprehensions and fears rising from astral forms they had "seen."

One class member had "seen" his mother standing by the fireplace as he sat reading one evening. He was still puzzling over the phenomenon when the telephone rang an hour later. This call informed him that his mother, involved in a car accident, was in the hospital but out of danger. The astral form he saw was a *telepathic apparition.*

Another class member told of visiting in a house where erratic occurrences were known to happen. During the night she was awakened by footsteps and "saw" a hooded figure move across the corner of her room. The experience shook her badly. She asked how protection from such astral phenomena could be demonstrated. The astral form she saw may have been an *apparition connected with the psychic record of the house.*

The nature of telepathic apparitions

It is a well-documented fact that during illness, in times of crisis or danger, and even in moments of great decision, a person's thoughts go out to those they cherish or back to places they love. Psychologically, the longing for communication with those you love may unconsciously draw you to them in moments of intense need, when the only way you can travel to them is by means of the astral body. It is this higher form of you that your loved one may see. This is what happened with the class member who "saw" his mother by the fireplace.

The astral body is free to move about and to convey its message as best it can. G. M. N. Tyrrell, explaining his theory of apparitions, says: "A telepathic apparition may, from one point of view, be regarded as a message expressed in the form of a three-dimensional picture . . . a moving picture."[4]

A similar emotional attachment to a *place,* rather than to a *person,* may provide the motive power that psychologically draws an individual back to the beloved surroundings of his childhood—to a place that provides psychic shelter. It is possible that a disinterested but sensitive stranger, now living in those cherished surroundings, may witness the fleeting form of an astral visitor.

Remember, in the account of Wilmot and Tait in their state-room on the high sea, Tait saw briefly an astral visitor who was a stranger to him. He had never met Mrs. Wilmot.

Although telepathic apparitions usually involve two people who are in rapport, this is not always the case. A stranger, in a quiescent mood or state of reverie, may tune into a level where the projected astral form of another person becomes visible.

Astral projection and so-called hauntings

What about the hooded figure seen by the class member in her bedroom? Astral forms from one source or another may very well account for so-called ghosts.

[4]Tyrell, G. N. M., *op. cit.,* p. 93, 96.

As explained in Chapter 4, everything that has transpired historically—everything that has been thought, experienced, and felt—leaves its subtle memory in the psychic record. In unexplained moments of attunement, a sensitive person may perceive this record. It may be as realistic as the ancient fair Miss Oliver "saw" that rainy afternoon she drove to Swindom in Wiltshire, England.

Many so-called ghosts may be apparitions perceived from the psychic record of a place—a house, a castle, a dungeon. The hooded figure seen by the class member may have been an impression stamped by a former tenant of the house in the psychic record—an impression imbedded by something intense that happened many years before. Intense emotions and events accompanying a crisis tend to leave a lasting psychic impression. These impressions repeat again and again like a video tape re-run time after time on TV.

This explanation is applicable for most so-called haunted houses. It is especially acceptable for phenomena which follow a pattern that becomes familiar for a specific house. Each spectator reports witnessing essentially the same episode.

But what of "ghosts" that seem to have a mind of their own? What of phenomena that follow no set pattern and are not simply re-runs from the psychic record?

Two other possibilities may be explored to furnish an explanation: One is the possibility that an apparition is the astral body of a living entity, illustrated by Tait's sighting of Mrs. Wilmot.

A second possibility is that the apparition is the astral body of a discarnate entity—the standard "ghost" of fiction and physical research. Far too many psychical apparitions, however, have been laid to the presence of a discarnate entity. The Science of Higher Sense Perception ascribes most apparations to astral projection in the form of telepathic apparitions, astral travel, and astral perceptions from the psychic record.

What is really there in apparitions?

"Does this mean," asked one student, "that in a haunted house the ghost is not really there?"

"What do you mean by *there*?"

"That the entity is not there—that it is only a mental picture."

To say something is *there* is to say that it occupies a certain position in space; it is a specific distance from one object or another; it is there where you can see it. But even when you are looking at someone in the flesh, you cannot actually say the person is *there* where you see him.

How often a person will remark of another, "I tried to talk with him but he was a million miles away!" He seemed to be there because his body was, but the real Self was not! Can it ever be said that the body is anything more than a *temporary* headquarters for the Self?

It is difficult to pin the real Self down, for it dwells in consciousness rather than in space. True, everybody's got to be someplace, but that someplace is at the point of one's awareness. You are where you are *aware* of being.

That awareness usually takes place where the body is, but, in deep thought, awareness may soar to interior heights or explore abroad by means of astral travel. It would be reasonable to assert that where your awareness is, *there* you are! Where another's awareness has taken him, *there* he is!

How to create a psychic shield of protection

Regardless of what is *there* or *not there*, it is a person's reaction to what he sees that can harm him or carry him safely through the encounter. The class member who saw the hooded figure in the corner of her room was badly frightened. Had she had a weak heart, the experience might have brought her serious harm.

Should she have refused her friend's invitation to spend the night in the house?

Should an owner, finding himself saddled with a "haunted" house, sell it—possibly sacrificing it at a loss?

What can you do for self-protection?

There is a way to protect yourself from undesirable psychic experiences, experiences that may bewilder you or disturb your peace of mind. There is a way to "lay any ghosts" you may encounter.

The whole principle of exorcism—practiced down through the centuries with a variety of weird techniques and ceremonies—involves the elements of belief and suggestion. The power of positive suggestion was administered by the witch doctor with incantations, it was administered by the minister with prayers and blessings, it was administered by the priest with the sign of the cross. *You can administer the power of positive suggestion through the commands you program into your subconscious mind.*

As you will find explained in more detail in the next chapter, things and places have a consciousness or aura all their own. If that aura is negative, you can subtly correct it through the positive quality of your own aura or consciousness.

In addition, you can build a psychic shield of protection around yourself that negative influences cannot pierce. To do this, use the Aura-of-Protection technique given you in Chapter 9.

Now, set the power of positive suggestion in motion by programming these commands into the subconscious mind: Command that all HSP encounters you have come as benefits and blessings. Affirm that nothing can enter your consciousness which is not beautiful, inspiring, and completely welcome. Command that nothing can influence your life that is not for your greater good. Then, use this Psi-Programming Pointer to keep yourself free of any fear that negative elements may invade your environment:

Ψ   Psi-Programming Pointer

THE POSITIVE QUALITY OF MY CONSCIOUSNESS INBUES MY HOME AND ENVIRONMENT WITH NEGATIVE-ERASING VIBRATIONS OF LOVE, POISE, POWER, FAITH, AND SERENITY.

Freeing yourself from environment influences

As you use the above psi-programming device, think of how the positive action of a magnet erases the previous program from an electronic tape replacing it with a new sound track. Like this, you can program into the subconscious mind new, positive vibrations and elements of attraction. You can erase negative vibrations from the psychic-record "tape." You need not be influenced by or continue to endure an undesirable "program."

The undesirable "program" connected with the classic haunted house may have been left on the psychic-record years before.

Sometimes an environment is haunted simply by the ill-wil' and unhappiness of those who live there currently. Sometimes it is inbued with negative impressions from the hatred or maliciousness of a past tenant. In any event, a negative environment is something you will wish to erase with new positive programming.

Many people are sensitive to the *feel* of a place. If it is cold and depressing, they may be feeling the chronic pessimism that a former owner impressed upon the psychic record there. If they feel a disquieting irritation, they may be sensing the hatred released by another tenant.

This is not to say that only *negative* elements are imprinted upon the psychic record by former tenants.

For example, a lady I know moved into a certain house. She knew nothing about it or its former occupants. As a young girl, she had studied music but had long since discontinued her lessons. After moving to her new address, she had a strong desire to study music again. She began taking lessons, and found great comfort and fulfillment in her music. Later, she learned that a well-known musician lived in the house before her.

This is not strange. It is entirely possible that the walls of the rooms still vibrated silently with harmony and that the psychic atmosphere resounded with music. The atmosphere influenced her subtly, without any conscious reason on her part, to cultivate again the musical talent deep within her.

It is possible for a house to be haunted in this sense. Undoubtedly, the strength of such impressions would depend upon the dynamic quality of the former tenant. A person with a strong and vital aura exudes a more lasting and permanent vibration. Strong beliefs, crisis situations, and emotionally-charged events are the stuff with which the psychic record of a place is built.

How to lay the "ghosts" of negation

Positive influences from the environment are, of course, something you do not have to protect yourself against. Regrettably, however, more negative influences seem to show themselves in the environment than constructive ones.

Hatred felt by those around one or by former dwellers seems to have a tenacious holding action. Hate holds a negative condition in place, whereas love releases it.

Quite possibly, the reason why so much phenomena in regard to apparitions is of a negative kind—centering around a house where someone was murdered or around some event of a tragic nature—is due to the holding and confining power of the negative. Hatred is confining while love is expansive. Hatred holds; love releases.

This gives us the clue to laying the ghost of negation. Be it the ghost of a cold, depressing environment or be it the classic "ghost" which "haunts" a locale as a visible apparition—whatever its purpose, nature, or function—the laying of the ghost is in release.

You can trigger that release through affirmations of love—a love that releases everyone to his greatest good. Specifically, use the Psi-Programming Pointer just given you to exercise the negative-erasing vibrations of love and serenity.

How HSP provides a protective armor

When astral phenomena are properly understood in terms of HSP principles, fears aroused by "haunted" houses, strange noises in the night, and apparitions, fade away.

What about other fears of the astral world?

Are you afraid that there are evil forces on the astral plane seeking to harm you here on the physical plane?

Can a so-called discarnate entity, looking for a body, displace your consciousness while you are sleeping or having an out-of-the-body experience?

Do you need protection from some mythical "they" from the astral world who would bring harm to you, usurp your will, and force you to do things you do not wish to do?

The Science of Higher Sense Perception answers such questions with an emphatic NO!

In the first place, the astral plane is as much your domain right now as the physical world. The *real you* is not your physical body, it is the invisible, permanent Self that created the body as its vehicle of expression. That Self finds the astral world as natural as the physical, although consciously you may not yet be aware of much beyond the physical.

No matter where the real Self is, it creates a *vehicle* of expression (physical or astral) out of the uniqueness of itself. Your physical body, from bone structure to finger prints, is tailored to the special person you are—there are no duplicates. Your physical body would "fit" no other consciousness. It is an extension of the real Self, an individualization of the *real you*. It can belong to no one else.

Your body reflects your thoughts, your feelings, your tendencies, your dominant self-image, your consciousness. This consciousness, built memory upon memory and experience upon experience, becomes a unique vibration. That unique vibration is *you*. Your body is a personalized expression of that uniqueness. There is no way for another person to possess your body, unless he is you.

You have *eminent domain*—first claim and absolute property rights! Your uniqueness makes your body your own, and you need never fear that it can be "possessed" by any other entity, carnate or discarnate. Besides, if there were such a thing as a homeless entity looking for a dwelling place, it would simply manifest its own vehicle of expression—for it is the nature of the real Self to do so!

But, you may ask, what of other possible evil astral forces? There *are* negative elements in the psychic record!

This is true. And when you feel depressed, moody, irritable, blue, resentful, angry, or apprehensive—for no obvious reason—it may mean that you have inadvertently tuned into a negative frequency on the lower psychic level. It may also mean that you have permitted your own consciousness to sink to a negative level in some regard. When you are resentful, you function on the plane where all vibrate who indulge in resentment. When your self-esteem falls to a low frequency, you function on the plane where all vibrate who indulge in self-pity and self-depreciation.

Therefore, it follows that the protection you need is not from something external to you. Your protection-need centers in your own consciousness. It is here you must work, raising your own vibration to a higher frequency—a frequency of self-esteem, faith, and love that turns negation away!

There is nothing down the road waiting to pounce on you as an unsuspecting traveler. The only thing that will ever pounce on you is the negation of your own mind or external negation to which you *permit* entry.

Programming protection into the subconscious

Feelings of security, strength, and self-confidence stem from a mind that develops the qualities discussed below. Study them and then work to assume them as your own. Program them into your subconscious mind with suggestion. Act "as if" they are yours, and your expectations will be fulfilled.

First, to build a psychic shield of protection, develop a mind that has *integrity*. Here integrity means *a state or quality of being complete, undivided, or unbroken*. It comes from the word *integer* meaning *a complete entity; especially, whole, not fractional*. In terms of higher sense perception, it denotes a mind that belongs to itself.

Such a mind is not vacillating, procrastinating, or swayed by every mass-consciousness wind that blows. It carefully evaluates every idea that comes to its attention. It retains ideas that add to its strength and wholeness. It dismisses any that would fracture that wholeness.

For example, you cannot hold two concepts that are incongruous. If you wish success for yourself, you cannot deny your neighbor success. If you wish friendship, you cannot perpetrate deceit and antagonism. This will shatter your mental integrity—your wholeness and invulnerability.

Second, to build your psychic armor, develop a keen sense of your *uniqueness*. Know that what belongs to you is yours and yours alone. Your body is an expression of your unique consciousness. It is a personalized expression of the real Self. It vibrates at a frequency unlike that of any other person who has ever lived! It fits no one else. It has its own psychic scent—peculiarly your own. It has been constructed by you and for you.

Only when the real Self no longer has *need* of the body will it lay it aside. When it *really* leaves the body, the physical building-blocks will disintegrate, for the psychic pattern within those blocks goes with you wherever you go!

Third, to build your psychic shield, enclose yourself in a circle of *love*. Remember, love releases all—all forces, all conditions, all entities—unto their greater good. In meditation, surround yourself and those who belong to you with love. Draw a mental circle around you, and let love radiate out from your heart to fill that circle. Love is a state of awareness in which no negative force can exist. Love turns aside ill-will, resentment, animosity, prejudice, and all man calls evil.

Love is never defeated. Should it seem to be, on observation it will be found that the shield of love has been lowered, or set aside, but never pierced. True love protects you from all harm.

Fourth, use HSP Sensitivity Training Technique No. 8 to unfetter yourself from any fears the astral world may have held for you. Use it to implement the instructions given you in this chapter.

HSP SENSITIVITY TRAINING TECHNIQUE NO. 8
YOUR PSYCHIC ARMOR OF PROTECTION

You are seated in your favorite chair and you begin by relaxing the various parts of your body. Starting with the feet, you move upward by consciously telling each part of the body, in turn, to relax. Your subconscious mind—in control of all autonomous bodily functions—is amenable to your conscious command and, through the involuntary nervous system, brings about the relaxation desired.

Now, you practice rhythmic breathing. Aware of your breath, you inhale deeply, counting to four slowly as you fill every cell of your lungs with air. Holding it for a count of four, you again count to four slowly as you expel all air from your body. On the final count, you wring out the last residue of air. Then, you repeat the process four times.

You sit now in quiet contemplation of the uniqueness of you. You realize that each tiny molecule is imbued with the special pattern which is you. Each cell is like the building-block of a vast temple that has been hewed by hand. This is the personalized temple of your body. The intricate design of your consciousness is wrought into the structure as if carved by a skilled artisan from individual specifications.

Those specifications can never be duplicated by another or possessed by another, for the secret of their creation lies in your own unique consciousness. No matter where you roam in this wide universe (physically or astrally), your body remains your own as long as you have need of it.

Maintaining this image of your own uniqueness, you surround the temple of the real Self with the radiant sunshine of love. Your body-temple is like a citadel bathed in the pure light of a fear-free love that emanates from your heart outward in a circle around you. You visualize that circle of love as a moat that turns away all that is unlike it—all that is unlovely, negative, or threatening. No harm can cross the moat and disturb the peace and poise of the dweller in the citadel.

Now, you strengthen your armor by eliminating anything threatening or discordant *within* your own consciousness. How do you accomplish this? By working for mental integrity, wholeness, and invulnerability. You program into your consciousness desires that do not clash with each other—desires that are compatible and congruous. You picture success for yourself, but a success that lets others prosper too. You see happiness for yourself, but not a selfish happiness that shows little true regard for others.

You visualize a protection for yourself that keeps you in good health and disposition. You visualize a protection for your business affairs that brings good fortune to them. You picture a protection for those close to you that assures their security and well-being.

You see yourself now, standing tall, strong, secure, serene, successful, and fear-free! You affirm silently, *"My life stands as a beacon of light, a tower of strength, and a citadel of security! I cannot be touched by negative forces, for only that which vibrates on a positive frequency can gain entry to my temple."*

(Abide in this feeling of safety and security for a few moments and then affirm:)

And so it is!

SUMMARY CAPSULES

HOW TO REGARD OUT-OF-THE-BODY SENSATIONS

Your body is not a container of you. It is simply a base of operations. It is home-plate for a Self that has the wide universe for its baseball diamond. The person who is not body-bound may find himself exploring the outfield, temporarily away from home base, in out-of-the-body sensations. The freedom to leave home-plate does not violate the rules of the game—rather, it indicates a game of much greater proportion!

HOW TO RETAIN CONSCIOUS COMMAND

There is nothing to fear about the experience-in-consciousness called astral projection, as long as the conscious mind retains the prerogative to start and end the phenomenon at will. Program your subconscious mind with the command that you experience nothing you do not *consciously* wish to experience! Command that you *deliberately* control your mind and all its HSP faculties!

HOW TO LAY A SO-CALLED GHOST

If you see an apparition, it very likely is an image you have lifted from the psychic record—an impression you get *visually* of some emotional event connected with a place. Or the apparition may be the astral form of a living or discarnate entity drawn to the place by some psychic bond. You may control such encounters by surrounding yourself with love, for love protects you and releases all that negation would hold in place.

HOW YOUR BODY BELONGS TO YOU

Your body is unique to you, for your consciousness has created it. Like custom-made shoes that conform to the peculiarities of your feet or a tailor-made suit cut specifically to your proportions, your consciousness has tailored your body to its uniqueness. Your tastes, talents, inclinations, and self-images are woven into the garment. No one else can "possess" it, for it fits the contours of your consciousness *only*.

9

How to Generate an Aura that Compels Success

Vivian was vivacious. This was the typical remark others made about her. The secret of her vivaciousness lay not entirely in her physical appearance. True, she was fairly attractive, but so are many thousands of other girls. Her attraction sprang from an invisible quality that she exuded with each movement, with each breath.

I had been making a study of auras—the energy-field that surrounds each person—when I first met Vivian. As she walked through the room, something strange appeared around her. Perhaps it was because of my preoccupation with auras and my interest in the subject that I witnessed what I did. As she moved toward me, I had the sensation of seeing a shimmering sheath or field of varicolored light accompanying her.

I thought my imagination was playing a trick on me, so I closed my eyes. When I opened them again, the intensity of her aura had dimmed somewhat. However, I could still see it, and it was real—to me. It was not, as a friend scoffed, "just due to the lighting in the room."

Everyone emanates an aura-lux

This was the first time I witnessed the aura of another person, an experience that has happened with varying degrees of intensity

175

ever since. It has demonstrated to me the fact that there is a vital field of energy surrounding each person. This field, sometimes visible as a shimmering lux or light, seems to influence the general success or failure of the individual. Vivian's aura-lux certainly brought her success and popularity.

There are those who radiate energy as freely as the sun warms the earth. There are others who walk through life in tightly locked cases of repressed energy. Those who are radiant have bright, scintillating auras. Thosy who are repressed have dull, lifeless auras. What makes the difference? The secret lies in enthusiasm, vitality, mental vigor, and thought intensity. I have seen people so enthusiastic about the ideas in which they believed that as they talked tiny shafts of light, radiating out from their silhouettes, were visible to me. Such people cannot help but be successful, for their enthusiasm compels success into their lives!

Now, a success aura need not be a visible emanation to be productive of good. Any positive degree to which your aura can be raised will bring desirable results into your life. Regardless of the color or intensity of your aura-lux at the present moment, you can generate a more positive emanation with the techniques given in this chapter.

How aura energy exerts control over things

It was 8:30 in the evening, and the HSP class I was conducting stopped for a coffee break. Auras had been the topic of the lesson just ended. I told them about Vivian and the aura energy-field emanating from each individual. "You may think of this emanation," I said, "as the energy-field of the real Self." When you are charged with enthusiasm over an idea, that field expands and becomes radiant. When you are cold to an idea, that field contracts. It may be compared to physical body heat. When you exercise enthusiastically, your body literally radiates heat that can be felt by others who are standing or sitting close to you. When you are physically cold, little body heat radiates from you. Little energy is generated.

Mental energy works similarly. For example, it is a common experience among those who shoot dice that when they generate a certain state they refer to as being "hot," they can radiate a degree of control over their tosses. Conversely, when they are "cold," lack of control is demonstrated.

Now if, when "hot," a dice player can actually influence the fall of an inanimate little cube of ivory, it means that some type of energy exists that radiates from his presence. It operates beyond the boundaries of his physical touch. This remote-control force springs from the aura energy of the real Self. Its reach is greater when enthusiasm and mental vigor are keen.

This ability of the real Self to control objects without physical contact has been called telekinesis or psychokinesis (PK). The action of PK, the mental movement of objects, explains many phenomena in addition to dice control. It underlies table tipping, ouija boards, levitation, slate writing, poltergeist, and the like.

As the class members sipped their coffee at the break, Frank, a salesman who had enrolled for the class, remarked, "I find it hard to believe that I can control the movement of objects with aura energy. When I want to move something, I use my hand like this," he asserted, shoving an ash tray across the snack bar counter.

"But, Frank," I said, "does your physical body actually have the ability to move objects by itself? Does an airplane actually have the power to move itself?" Frank raised his eyebrows quizzically as I went on to explain: Power is what energizes material form. The aircraft itself is inanimate without the fuel that propels it. The plane is not energy itself. It uses energy. The physical form cannot act without the mental energy that vitalizes it. The body is not energy itself. It uses energy.

The mind is the real power. It is the moving power behind all life. It, however, is the element frequently overlooked when science examines energy. The science of energetics has dealt with *energy* from the standpoint of its conversion, its transformation, its conservation, and its indestructability. But *energy itself* eludes the scientist who must think of it in terms of matter. Energy is not what is expressed. It is the cause of expression. And the *cause* is always greater than the mode through which it expresses. Hence, energy transcends the form. It transcends the body. It transcends the aircraft.

"Frank," I said, "remember that you are not a body that has a mind, but a mind that has a body. The real Self is something greater than the body. In the same way, you are not a body that expresses energy. You are energy that expresses through a body. Thus, when you moved the ash tray just now, it was the energy of the real Self that moved it. The physical body served merely as a vehicle through which the real Self acted."

When you are charged with enthusiasm and mental vigor, the energy of the real Self radiates *beyond* the confines of the physical body. This radiation is your aura. It is your psychokinetic energy. If you wish, think of it as the energy that may be exerted by the real Self through your astral body. Or, very simply, think of it as the power of mind over matter.

Practical benefits of building a positive aura

The potentialities of the mind-over-matter theory have been studied in the parapsychology lab with experiments in dice rolling. The fall of dice has been utilized as a device for testing psycho-kinetic energy, for theoretically physical skill cannot influence the outcome. Controlled experiments have been carried on involving one die thrown from the hand or a cup, pairs of dice released from rotating cages, and combinations of 4, 6, 8, and more dice. Tests have involved the calling of one face of the die, or a combination of numbers, or high die, or low die.

J. B. Rhine, who has carried on extensive scientifically-con-trolled PK tests, reports that his experiments yield results suffi-ciently above chance to be interesting and concludes that something other than chance is operating.

Incidentally, the method Rhine employed in testing for PK was suggested to him by a young gambler. As Rhine writes:

> This young man had visited the Duke Laboratory to discuss what he considered the role of ESP in gambling practices. He also asserted stoutly his confident belief that he could mentally influence the fall of dice under the right conditions and accepted the challenge to demon-strate the point. He succeeded well enough to justify a thorough test of his claims; he called it, "The Law of Mind over Matter."[1]

It was Frank talking again: "What bothers me," he said, "is the question of what *value* all this is to me personally. So the mind

---
[1]Rhine, Joseph Banks, *New World of the Mind.* New York: William Morrow & Co., Inc., 1953, p. 38.

can influence the roll of dice! I'm not a gambler, and I don't shoot dice. Of what practical benefit is the mental movement of objects, assuming that I could even develop the ability?"

I understood Frank's attitude. He was a salesman. Practical techniques were what he wanted to improve his sales quotas and personal measure of success. What I had said about auras and psychokinetic energy was interesting to him, but he wanted to know how to relate this to his life and work.

"Frank," I said, "I know you are not a gambler. But you do play cards, and I'll bet you never pass up the chance to cut the pack when the dealer next to you has shuffled. In a sense, you are cutting your own consciousness into the game when you cut the deck."

A person's aura makes its effects felt in subtle ways whether he is selling cars, rolling dice, or playing cards. If an individual has a winning streak, the cards seem to fall into a general pattern that enables the individual to win. He may call it luck, but a subtle telekinetic force is involved. It is an expression of his winning consciousness. On the other hand, if an individual has a losing consciousness—a negative aura—that person will tend to lose when playing cards. In the game of life, as in a card game, a losing consciousness will influence things and people to react negatively.

"Frank," I explained, "you cannot do anything from cutting a deck of cards to investing on the stock exchange without subtly influencing life either positively or negatively toward you according to your consciousness-aura. As a salesman, your aura reaches out beyond the confines of your body to influence the reaction of people toward you. Your attitude subtly determines whether sales develop in your favor or not. In the business field, you are always walking ahead of your physical self. The distinctive atmosphere of your aura steps into the presence of others before you shake their hands—conditioning their response to you. What you need now are the mechanics of building an aura that will make your telekinetic potentialities positive and constructive."

Frank nodded in agreement, and we finished the last of our coffee. Here is what I told Frank and the HSP class members as they settled themselves in their seats for the second portion of the lesson following our conversation at coffee break. Here, too, are the principles you can apply to build a positive aura that compels success.

How your aura aids in the attainment of success

A dictionary definition of *aura* furnishes an excellent springboard for its study: *1. Any subtle, invisible emanation or exhalation; 2. A distinctive atmosphere surrounding a person; 3. ELEC.: A draft, or motion of the air caused by electric repulsion, as when the air near a charged metallic point is set in motion.*

Basically, an aura is a subtle, normally invisible emanation of energy—an energy-atmosphere surrounding a person. It reflects the measure of intensity at which the Self functions at the moment. Its lux or light grows more radiant with enthusiasm and wanes with discouragement.

Generally, the aura is colored by the overall consciousness of the individual. In other words, your aura is distinctly your own. It is as distinct to the *mental you* as your scent is to the *physical you.* Your aura seems to permeate your possessions and imbue the things you handle with your particular uniqueness (the basis upon which psychometry is premised.)

Your consciousness clings to your possessions as tenaciously as your scent clings to your clothing. It identifies you. Impossible? Not when you consider that even your physical scent is so tenacious and unique that it remains, at least temporarily, upon the ground where you have walked. A dog trained for tracking, given one of your shoes to sniff, can pick out and follow your unique physical emanation along the path you walked hours before.

Your mental aura is even more powerful than your physical scent, although the physical can sometimes be quite overpowering. The body odor and bad breath ballyhooed in TV commercials are no joke. An offensive physical odor may very well cause failure in the business and social world. However, the handicap of an undesirable breath or perspiration odor is easy enough to overcome because it is readily detectable. By contrast, a negative aura, more powerful than any physical emanation, is felt by others only in subtle ways. Your best friend—as the ad-men depict it—may give you a bottle of gargle to freshen your breath, but that same friend will not be able to detect a negative aura as readily. He will simply feel depressed and uncomfortable in your presence and excuse himself as soon as possible.

If failure, lack of friends, and poor luck seem to plague you, you can generally assume that your aura is negative. As pointed out before, man's aura is colored by his overall consciousness. It is the emanation of his self-image. If he is self-deprecating, defensive, belligerent, overly-aggressive, fault-finding, opinionated, acutely ego-centered, or filled with self-pity, this will lend a negative hue to his aura that others will feel. Friends will be repelled by such negative emanations and success will be turned aside.

What can you do to overcome a negative aura? Use the comprehensive HSP sensitivity-training technique given at the end of this chapter to correct and improve your aura. During the day, however, when there is no quiet time for this formal training, repeat the following short psi-programming pointer:

Ψ   Psi-Programming Pointer
MOMENT BY MOMENT, I BUILD AN AURA WHICH RADI-
ATES POSITIVE QUALITIES THAT OTHERS FIND ATTRAC-
TIVE, AN AURA THAT COMPELS A RESPONSE OF GOOD
WILL AND GOOD FORTUNE.

The effect of your aura-atmosphere on others

Whenever you come into the presence of another person, your aura reacts with his. This reaction is the basis for so-called snap-judgment. Can snap-judgment be relied upon; is it correct? It is correct only in this way: If you instantly dislike someone upon first meeting, it may tell you that he is negative or wrong for you as a friend. On the other hand, it may tell you that there is something negative or discordant in your own consciousness at the moment which clashes with the aura of the person you have just met.

At any rate, it is the reaction of your aura with the aura of others as you come together that turns you on or off. When you are with certain people, you feel vital and energized. Their aura-atmosphere seems to excite and stimulate your own energy field. There may be other people who deplete your emotional and mental resources and leave you limp physically.

Some individuals are virtual "sappers." They drain the vitality of those around them. It is a strain to be with them and to ward off their negative aggression, criticism, and demands. In a way, they are *psychic vampires;* they feed upon the strength of others. If you are in their presence for a prolonged period, you become de-energized. If auras were as obvious as body odor, it would be no trick to detect the negative aura of a "sapper," but a negative consciousness is subtle. It can be detected, however, by its effects on you. If being with someone leaves you as limp as a rag, you can feel assured that negative elements are present.

Have you ever remarked after a trying visit with an acquaintance, "Just talking to him makes me tired!" or, "She takes so much out of me!"? If you have had this experience with someone repeatedly, that person is not one you will wish to cultivate. Of course, if he is a relative or business associate with whom you must come in contact, you can protect yourself through the toning of your own aura. You can raise your own consciousness to the point where no negative outside element can penetrate it. To do this, use the next psi-programming pointer that is given in this chapter.

It sometimes happens in marriage that one partner, with constant demands and excessive needs, will sap the mental and emotional strength of the second partner. The second mate may feel depleted for years without ever suspecting the cause of the exhaustion. However, quite the opposite is often the case. One n arriage partner may vitalize the other by his mere presence. Each mate then mutually prospers from the scintillating and harmonious *interaction* of compatible aura-atmospheres.

The success aura in marriage and business

In a successful marriage, the aura of husband and wife vibrate synchronously together. They feel good in each other's presence. Harmonious functioning is vital to success, peace of mind, understanding, rapport, and happiness. On the other hand, where auras clash, a negative reaction is set in motion that can drive from the marriage happiness, compatibility, and even financial adequacy.

In a successful business, this same aura-synchronization exists. This is why some partnerships prosper while others fail. On the surface, successful business partners may be quite different in personality and disposition. Yet from the standpoint of their aura energy-fields, they prove to be harmonious. They synchronize together with positive elements of compatibility. They are supportive of each other. The ideas, ideals, and purposes of one augment the other. Using HSP techniques, you can be guided into the company of a marriage partner or business partner with whom you are compatible. You can also demonstrate protection from the jarring effects of people in your environment with negative auras.

As you work with the laws of higher sense perception, you will become aware of the quality of another person's aura-atmosphere and be able to modify its effect upon you. This is what Frank learned to do. It was less than a month after he started using the sensitivity training technique for building a success aura which I gave the class that Frank had results to report.

"Before going out to make my sales contacts," Frank declared, "I've learned to sit down and generate an aura that is positive. I visualize a lux of sincerity, friendliness, honesty, and genuine regard for my customers' best interests radiating from me. I picture prospects *feeling* that radiance even before I shake their hands. And it's worked wonders for me! People have become a hundred percent more responsive. My sales performance is soaring!

"Of course, I still run into prospects who are negative and unfriendly. But, I've found that I can raise my own aura to compensate for their lack of response. The moment I feel their resistance, I increase my own enthusiasm. Not that I become pushy," Frank hastened to add, "but I generate an inner faith in my product that others feel. And, my product just seems to sell itself!"

Frank found for himself the secrets of a success aura that you are now uncovering. Whatever field of endeavor you wish to succeed in or whatever personal relationship you wish to improve, the building of a more positive aura will aid you in your attainment.

Use HSP Sensitivity-Training Technique No. 9 to build a strong, glowing, independently vigorous aura of your own. If you detect that you have been drawing upon the strength of others or that others have been leaning upon your strength, work to protect yourself right now with the following Psi-Programming Pointer. Use this programming device to declare protection for yourself and to build an awareness of personal power.

Ψ   Psi-Programming Pointer

I AM NOT A LEANER, NOR AM I LEANED UPON. MY AURA IS STRONG, VITAL, AND VIGOROUS IN MY OWN RIGHT AS AN INDEPENDENT CENTER OF UNIVERSAL MIND.

Psychometry—a ramification of aura energy

The ramifications of the aura man builds and emanates are many. As pointed out, this aura is tenacious. It seems to cling to man's very possessions, even as his scent remains as a smell which a bloodhound may track. Indeed, this "scent" aspect of an aura is demonstrated by the phenomena produced through psychometry.

Psychometry is defined as *the divination of facts concerning an object or its owner through contact with, or proximity to, the object.* A person who is sensitive psychically is frequently able to take an object in his hand and identify its owner or perceive the general history of the article.

A certain fortune teller uses this ability as a device to delight her clientele. Upon entering the hall, each visitor is requested to leave on a table an object belonging to him—a cigarette lighter, a handkerchief, etc. At a point in the program, the psychic takes each article in turn and holds it in her hand. Concentrating, she is frequently able to identify its owner by his initials and give some facts about his occupation, his marital status, and the like.

Is the object she holds literally imbued with some mental "scent" from its owner? Does an aura actually cling to it, or does the psychic use the object merely to attune telepathically with its owner? To a degree, both possibilities apply.

Telepathy is certainly involved—in which case the object serves as a focal point or "dial" for the tuning of one mind to another on the level of higher sense perception. It is possible, too, that the aura of the owner clings to or modifies in some subtle way the magnetic field of the object.

How can this be? Every inanimate object is a unique magnetic field of energy corresponding to its molecular structure. The structure of each element is distinct; each has its own atomic weight and vibratory uniqueness. Scientists can measure these unique magnetic fields. They exist! They are real!

A quartz rock, with an adequate measuring device, could be depicted as a magnetic field of a certain quality and intensity. A cigarette lighter, again with a suitable measuring device, could be depicted as a different magnetic field with its own characteristics.

The magnetic field of an object such as a lighter may be modified to a degree by the handling of its owner. Perhaps the modification in vibration would be temporary—like a scent which grows weaker with the elapse of time.

At any rate, an object *does* seem subject to modification by the positive or negative aura of its possessor. This principle partly explains the so-called power of an object that is "cursed." It partly explains the efficacy of good-luck charms and artifacts that are said to bring good fortune. The theory of carrying an amulet that has been blessed rests on this premise.

The other half of the explanation rests on the power of belief. The good-luck charm brings fortune to its owner partly because of his *belief* in it. The "cursed" object has the power to jinx its owner mainly because of his *fear* of it. The lucky hat, the old tie, or beloved shoes worn by the actor to assure success on opening night bring good fortune in proportion to his *faith* in them.

How to break a jinx

There is no reason to let an object that is reputedly cursed or a possession that is rumored to be jinxed have any power over you. Whether the source of the jinx lies in your own fear or in some negative modification of the magnetic field of the thing itself, you have the power to right it. You can right your fear by placing an aura of protection around yourself that screens out all threats and leaves you unharmed and strong. You can cancel any negative vibration with which an object seems inbued with your own positive mental state.

How do you create this AURA OF PROTECTION? You simply program a *protection-command* into your consciousness. Primarily, it is a mental act. To make that act dramatic and compelling, take these steps.

1. Assume a meditative state, becoming quiet, poised, and self-confident.

2. Remember that the real Self is something greater than the body. It rules the body as commander-in-chief.

3. Now, draw an invisible circle around yourself with your arms outstretched. Begin by touching the tips of your fingers together in front of you. Slowly swing your arms out to the sides and then behind you, completing the circle as the tips of your fingers touch behind you.

4. As you draw this invisible circle with your arms, *mentally* encircle yourself with an aura. Picture the aura as a golden lux that glows around you. See it growing brighter and purer. This light is your consciousness. It is positive, constructive, creative, success-prone, powerful, beneficient, and healthful! Its radiance repels anything unlike it.

5. Now, with the authority of the real Self, declare protection for yourself, repeating the words of the following psi-programming pointer three times. Reaffirm this consciousness-programming declaration when necessary, to keep your mental state strong. Your positive aura-lux will repel any negative force or influence that comes into your range of experience. It dispels it as surely as darkness disappears when the light is turned on.

Ψ   Psi-Programming Pointer

I NOW SURROUND MYSELF WITH AN AURA OF PRO-
TECTION. THAT AURA GLOWS WITH POSITIVE QUALITIES
OF GOOD FORTUNE, HEALTH, SUCCESS, AND GOOD WILL.
NOTHING NEGATIVE CAN PENETRATE ITS PROTECTIVE
CIRCLE.

Poltergeist—a phenomenon of excess aura energy.

Still another ramification of man's aura energy-field points toward the phenomena referred to popularly as poltergeist. In the realm of unexplained mysteries, peculiar happenings have been reported such as falling pebbles, knockings, voices, mischievous movement of household objects, pranks with walls that squirt water, trickery with undialed telephones that ring, and the like. These unsolved riddles seem to involve dematerialization, rematerialization, teleportation, and a host of science-fiction type manifestations.

For lack of a scientific explanation, such phenomena have often been attributed to a *polter* (noisy) *geist* (ghost)—a term of German-French origin. The name suggests that these mysteries are of spirit origin, the work of one returned from the dead. However, new evidence now implies that poltergeist phonomena are very much the work of the living.

Curiously, when poltergeist activity appears, it is almost invariably in a household where a young person is present or someone who has a capricious or dual personality. C. G. Jung mentions this significant point in his volume entitled *The Archetypes and the Collective Unconscious:*

> It is not surprising to find certain phenomena in the field of parapsychology which remind us of the trickster. These are the phenomena connected with poltergeists, and they occur at all times and places in the ambience of preadolescent children. [2]

Since Jung's pronouncement, many researchers in parapsychology have confirmed the likelihood that a young person may become the inadvertent agent for poltergeist manifestation. I say *inadvertent,* because the one responsible for the manifestation is primarily unconscious of the media through which his excess energy is expressing.

A case of classic poltergeist manifestations

Here is a typical case involving a family with a young daughter. It is reported by Hans Bender, M.D., Ph.D., a German psychiatrist who directs a team of researchers at the Institute for Border Areas of Psychology and Mental Health of Freiberg University:

> Beginning in November, 1968, and continuing for four months, poltergeist phenomena began in an almost classical way at the home of

---

[2] Jung, Carl G., *The Archetypes and The Collective Unconscious.* Bollingen Series XX, Vol. 9, Part 1. Princeton: Princeton University Press, 1959, p. 256.

the Redl family. The focus of the phenomena was the 13-year old daughter, Brigitte. There were knocks on the windows and doors. Stones rained on the house and later even penetrated inside, though the doors and windows were closed.

When a priest was brought in to bless the house against the "demons," a stone fell from the ceiling at that very moment. It landed on the wooden board of a cabinet but, curiously, did not bounce. When the priest picked it up, it felt warm.

The next stage began when the little girl's dolls and knick-knacks began flying about the room, sometimes even around corners. Linen appeared mysteriously from closed closets. Eggs cracked in visitors' hats, and less humorously, their coats were shredded.[3]

Bender and his team of researchers were called in to investigate the mystery. They put objects in locked cases and set cameras to trip if anything occurred. Subsequently when they were all outside, the lights in the house suddenly switched on. They rushed back in and checked the boxes. They found that a figurine in one of the locked cases had fallen over in the box. However, the light curtain had not been broken to trip the camera.

"This event was hardly explainable by normal causes and could suggest some initial PK endeavors to displace the figure,"[4] declares Bender. He further comments that even if the figurine had been found outside the box, he would scarcely have expected the photoelectric light curtain to have responded. Obviously, Bender feels that what takes place in such phenomena is above ordinary sense perception. It is HSP phenomena.

What psychokinetic principles are involved in poltergeist?

Earlier in this chapter it is pointed out that a person's aura or *consciousness-emanation* reaches out beyond the confines of his body to influence the reaction of people and objects around him. The energy of his aura, as a psychokinetic or telekinetic force, is a power that he can direct (as in the roll of dice when a player is *hot.*) When psychological pressures build up in the personality, there is a possibility that the telekinetic energy of the aura goes on a rampage. It exerts telekinetic force in non-directed ways.

---

[3]Vaughan, Alan, "Poltergeist Investigations in Germany," *Psychic.* Vol. 1, No. 5, March-April, 1970, p. 11-12.

[4]*Ibid.,* p. 13.

This force behaves capriciously, carrying on mischievous and even malicious telekinetic pranks that bring its owner a degree of psychological release from pressure. It is felt by parapsychologists that among the pressures which cause these uncontrolled bursts of aura-activity are unhappiness, resentment, and frustration—states that may become quite acute in the child and adolescent. These pressures produce a paranormal extension of normal abilities, resulting in non-directed HSP phenomena.

In exploring this aspect of the aura, consider again one of the definitions given earlier in this chapter. An *aura,* electrically, is described as being *a draft, or motion caused by electric repulsion, as when the air near a charged metallic point is set in motion.* The aura of the individual *is* a magnetic or electrical field of energy. It may be said that when this field becomes over-charged with rebellion, unhappiness, resentment, or frustration, motions near it become erratic. These motions constitute a psychic storm.

Perhaps a young person is more susceptible to this over-charged state, for in a growing child the cell population of the body expands rapidly. The magnetic aura-field expands correspondingly fast, generating excess energy not yet harnessed for the creative pursuits of adulthood. If for some reason the child is then exposed to undue tensions, inner rebellion and frustration may build up and express as unconscious, uncontrolled poltergeist manifestations. Similar tensions in an adult at times of stress and anxiety may result, too, in these psychic "electrical" storms—accounting for unexplained noises, movement of objects, and the like. It may be postulated that poltergeist are the thunder and lightning of aura-energy (psychokinetic energy), exploding under a build-up of psychological tensions.

The subject of poltergeist, of course, is too complex and profound to be fully explored in a few short paragraphs. However, the *aura energy-storm* theory advanced by the Science of Higher Sense Perception satisfactorily explains much that is classified as poltergeist phenomena.

How to eliminate the "geist" in poltergeist

An uncontrolled electrical storm can cause great damage. Lightning created by it may burn a house down; a booming clap of thunder may start a landslide. Unharnessed power is unpredictable. Today man has learned to harness electrical power, using it to turn mighty turbines, to light his cities, and to drive the wheels of industry. This is channeled power. It is predictable and useful.

Just as man has learned to discipline electrical power and harness it for his use, the individual can learn to direct and control the psychokinetic power of his aura energy to make it predictable and useful. This control can be gained through the exercise of the power of suggestion. To control aura energy is to harness it, not to suppress it. It may be channeled into constructive uses and become a force-for-good in the world rather than a source of mischief.

It has been demonstrated that *suggestion* and *expectation* play a vital role in the occurrence of poltergeist activity. A family in Lawrence, Massachusetts, in 1967, was plagued with jets of water exploding unexplicably from the walls of the house. Of the phenomenon, it was reported that the witnesses caught on to the rhythm of the manifestation and

> When the witnesses had seen an explosion on one wall, they would expect another on another wall. And they were not disappointed . . . When a few bubbles were noticed on furniture, the spectators would talk as if they expected more, and their predictions were fulfilled in a few minutes.[5]

Certainly, if suggestion can increase poltergeist activity, it can decrease it and eliminate it. According to Raymond Bayless, author of *The Enigma of the Poltergeist*, the power of suggestion is a logical tool to use in the exorcising of poltergeist: "Inasmuch as the birthplace of the poltergeist is found within the unconscious then the key to controlling this force through exorcism is suggestion."[6]

The key to control is, without a doubt, in the power of suggestion. The key to improving your aura—making it more radiant, channeling its psychokinetic energy to positive and creative ends, raising its brilliance to attract success to you—lies in your conscious ability to program your subconscious mind with mental commands.

---

[5] Bayless, Raymond, *The Enigma of the Poltergeist*. New York: Parker Publishing Co., 1967, p. 93-94.

[6] *Ibid.*, p. 177.

Steps to generate an aura that compels success

Here are the conscious steps you may take to generate an aura that compels success. These steps deal with qualities of mind you must deliberately cultivate. Remember, the subconscious mind responds to your conscious suggestion and expectation, so court these qualities *fully expecting* them to intensify your aura along positive lines.

First, cultivate belief: Belief precedes all real accomplishment. Nothing of a worthwhile nature can be achieved without it. If there is some reason why you should *not believe* you are greater than you thought before picking up this book, if there is some reason why you should *not believe* you possess untapped and unused powers of mind—powers you should be radiating with every word you utter and breath you draw—I am at a loss to know what that reason might be, other than your prior conditioning. Reject self-limitations! Reject stingy expectations! Reject narrow *prior beliefs* that have programmed your mind up to now!

There is no scientific reason for not believing in a greater you. There is no reason for not believing in personal success! Believe in your greater Self and in the powers potential to it. Belief will awaken the sleeping giant within you!

Second, cultivate desire: Intensify your desire to know more about yourself. Desire the rich gifts of life! However, let your first desire be for greater wisdom.

Don't let your yearning for wisdom be idle day-dreaming. Be up and doing! Desire which is dynamic goes *to work* to accomplish its ends. Your desire must be so intense that you feel you cannot wait another day to know and to be your greater Self.

This intensity, however, must be accompanied by the calm, poised assurance that what you desire will be demonstrated. A farmer may desire a crop of corn, but his desire will be on its way to fulfillment *only* when he releases it to the soil by sowing "seed corn." Desire greatly, but then release your "desire seed" and let life demonstrate it.

Third, cultivate enthusiasm: Remember Vivian? Her aura fairly scintillated with enthusiasm and mental vitality. The player who is *hot* is vibrant with the excitement of enthusiasm. Emerson, speaking of enthusiasm, says that "nothing great has ever been accomplished without it."

Enthusiasm is the generator that expands the radiance of your aura-lux, stepping up the frequency of your energy and expanding the radius of your influence. The word *enthusiasm* comes from the Greek *en (in) theos (God),* and literally means *in a divine state; in inspiration; possessed by inspiration.*

To be enthusiastic for life—to be vibrant with an idea—is to become like a magnet. Its invisible influence is felt at a distance. Its power performs feats of accomplishment. It draws its own unto itself.

Fourth, cultivate empathy and love: Love expands, while selfishness contracts. To expand the aura of your consciousness, cultivate a deep and sincere interest in other people and genuine appreciation for all creation. Love is a universal feeling. It generates understanding and empathy—the ability to participate in the viewpoint of others.

Love and empathy are essential to the intensification of your aura and its constructive use. Love for mankind keeps your aura positive and makes it a force-for-good in the world. An aura that radiates love can bring no harm to its owner or to those around him.

Fifth, cultivate a sensitivity or awareness of the potentialities of your real Self through the systematic HSP Sensitivity Training Technique that follows. This training gives you a technique for developing all the aura-expansion and aura-control factors explained in the chapter.

HSP SENSITIVITY-TRAINING TECHNIQUE NO. 9

EXPANDING YOUR SUCCESS AURA

You are seated in the chair you reserve for your meditative HSP sensitivity training. With your eyes closed, you relax each muscle as you have learned to do in previous chapters. Finally, you become aware only of your awareness.

You raise your attention now to the center of your forehead. In occult teachings, this is the third-eye position. You visualize a light located in this position. This light, at first a small glow inside the forehead, begins to expand within you. It is a radiance that spreads from the front of your head backward to the base of your skull. It then moves downward, illumining every corner of your inner body.

You continue, in your imagination, to feel the presence of this light inside you. You *suggest* that it glows brighter, purer, and more vibrant. You *expect* it to do so! Your expectations are rewarded. Your whole inner world now seems aglow with your radiant aura-light.

Then you mentally draw an outer circle around you and let your aura shine outward through the third-eye—that point between and above your closed eyes. Your aura now fills the circle around you with a radiant light. That light is the glow from your consciousness.

You now program into your consciousness your desires for good fortune, success, creativeness, achievement, and constructive service to your world. How do you do it? You visualize your desires! You vitalize your desires with enthusiasm! You inspire yourself with your desires! The more inspiration you generate, the more your aura-lux glows!

Now you visualize others walking into the radiance of your aura. See them smile as they approach you. See them reach favorably toward you. Visualize successful responses resulting from their positive reaction to your good will, empathy, and love. See your aura going before you as you step out into the world of business, finance, friendship, and marriage—assuring you relationships that bless you and those with whom you come in contact.

(Read this sensitivity-training technique several times, until you can follow it mentally in your own words with your eyes closed. Tailor it to your own specific desires, keeping them positive and dynamic. Repeat it daily for a week, to increase the results. Believe deeply now—and every time you use this training—that your aura is expanding with each meditation. Mentally draw an ever-widening circle of light around you, until your aura reaches out to bless all mankind.)

You remain, now, in the awareness of the inner and outer glow experienced in this session as your mind becomes quiet. You feel a calm, poised assurance of new radiance, new power, new vivaciousness! You close, when ready, affirming:

And so it is!

SUMMARY CAPSULES

HOW TO BUILD A POSITIVE AURA

The degree of success or failure you experience depends upon the *aliveness* of the energy field surrounding you. This field is an expression of your consciousness. It is your aura! To assure success, work to build an aura that is *alive* and *positive* with constructive ideas, exciting plans, enthusiasm, imagination, and creative self-images. A positive aura compels success into your life!

HOW TO LIFT YOUR ENTHUSIASM-QUOTIENT

An aura is like the atmosphere around a planet—as warm and pulsating with life as Earth or as cold and lifeless as the Moon. Make your aura pulsate with new energy by raising your enthusiasm-quotient! How? Make plans you can feel intense about. Pursue things that spark you with inspiration. Get "hot" with the idea of achievement. And watch your aura pulsate with the vibrant atmosphere of a "live" planet!

HOW YOUR AURA-ATMOSPHERE AFFECTS OTHERS

When your aura interacts with another's, you may find a response that is harmonious, neutral, or discordant. In the latter case, the reaction may be due to negative elements in the other's consciousness or in your own. Regardless, you can control the reaction and its affect upon you by raising your own consciousness to compensate. A higher consciousness changes you, changes the other person, or changes the interaction between you.

HOW TO INVOKE YOUR PSYCHOKINETIC POWER

To a subtle degree, the aura of magnetic energy surrounding you constantly influences people and things in your world. The force it exerts is your psychokinetic power. PK is an invisible force that is invoked by your enthusiasm and mental vigor. It is directed by your conscious (or more frequently, unconscious) suggestion. It is so much a part of you that you seldom recognize its role in your exercise of mind over matter.

HOW TO STILL POLTERGEIST "STORM" PHENOMENA

Uncontrolled mental energy is like power unleashed in a storm. It is "lightning" that may spark, crackle, and pop in erratic ways. The uncontrolled aura energy of a young person *under tension* may explode unconsciously as "psychic storm" phenomena. Later, as an adult, he usually channels this energy into positive endeavors. Meanwhile, through HSP Sensitivity Training, a young person can come to understand himself and how to control his powers.

10

How to Reach Beyond
This Present Time and Place

"Do you believe in reincarnation?" Karen asked. "Do you feel that we have lived before? Does life continue beyond this time and place?"

"Slow down a bit with the questions," I said to my visitor, "and tell me first why you are interested in reincarnation."

"Well," Karen replied, "I'm thrilled with the results I have been getting with your sensitivity training techniques, but sometimes as I become quiet and relaxed, I get odd *flashback* impressions."

"What are they like?"

"Actually," Karen explained, "since childhood I've gotten them—sometimes as dreams, sometimes as day-dreams. In my twenties, they came less frequently and only when I was in a state of reverie. Now, they have happened twice during HSP training."

She continued, "The flashback is like watching a movie on TV and having another channel cut in. The scenes are not related to my present life, yet they seem to involve me intimately."

"For instance?" I queried.

"Well," my visitor said, "the flashbacks are essentially the same as a recurring dream I had when I was a child. It is a scene of myself when I am five or six years of age. There are two other children, and a man and woman. We are in a cabin along a stream. There is a storm, and the water rises around the cabin. I see the man, who seems to be my father, struggling to save us. But, the cabin is swept away, and suddenly there is nothing except blackness."

"I feel strongly," Karen declared, "that a previous incarnation for me ended in such a manner. Of course, I'll concede that other explanations for my dream are possible."

A personal case of psychic-record dreaming

Karen looked at me rather quizzically, as if half-expecting me to explain her feelings away. Instead, I shared with her a personal experience that I have related before to only a few kindred people.

When I was about eighteen, I had an unusually vivid dream. By vivid, I am not referring to the garishness of a nightmare, but to the clarity that involves deep-memory perception.

I found myself in a far-away region that was strange to me—strange after I awoke from the dream. However, during it I felt a perfect sense of belonging. The terrain I beheld was different from the rolling hills and forest land of West Virginia, which was my home. The dream-scene was of grassy, level, prairie land.

In my dream I saw a house that I knew to be my home in this flat, open country. There were vivid, distinguishing features about the house—its placement on the land, how the road turned sharply around the corner of the house, details of design, the stately old lines, the porches, the fence. There was a large tree growing across the road to the south of the house. The dream was most intense. The impressions it left with me were most forceful and realistic.

A short time after this dream, I left West Virginia. Although my intended destination was California, I paused for a time on my journey in Ohio and Illinois. I had long since forgotten about my dream which, by now, had occurred about four years before.

Circumstances then brought me as far west as Denver, Colorado. I went to the North Park area for a summer and, in the fall, started back to Denver with a friend. Our route took us through Greeley. *There,* I saw my house! A strong feeling arose in me that I had been there before, and then I remembered my dream!

It was the same stately old house, the same road, the same distinctive features I had seen in my dream! I had the feeling of coming home. The impulse to go into the house was intense, but I felt my companion would have thought it strange so I resisted the urge. Besides, I could think of no logical reason for doing so at the time. I shrugged off the incident, and we continued our trek to

Denver. In the months to follow, however, I thought again and again about that house and the enigma of my dream. At that time, I had no answer to the riddle.

Perhaps the dream was clairvoyant—I simply had "seen" in the dream-state a place I was to see in person four years hence. Or, perhaps the dream was a composite—a subjective synthesis—of places I had visited and pictures I had seen in books. Or, perhaps the feeling I had that day on the road to Greeley was simple wishful thinking—maybe a desperate longing to be home again called back the long forgotten vision.

However, I think not! None of these explanations fit my feeling as the dreamer. That house had been my home one time!

As explained in Chapter Seven, dreams are one medium through which impressions may arise from the deep-memory record of the psychic level—a level where images of yesterday, yesteryear, and yesterlives are stored. In the dream state, *regression flashes* of a previous life are logical phenomena.

Regression to childhood is not at all uncommon under hypnosis. Regression also occurs at times during serious illness and mental derangement when the subconscious is dominant. In psychological experiments with memory regression during hypnosis, valid evidence of former lives has been produced, indicating that a deep-memory record exists and may be tapped.

If the psychic life of man is continuous, then doors to previous living may become slightly ajar or may at times swing wide, permitting a glimpse into a previously-occupied room in the House-of-Self. It is no mystery that the experiences of a former life, stored away in an individual's personal psychic record, may arise as impressions which find their way to the surface. This, I feel, was true of my dream and of Karen's flashbacks.

"In a former life, I was Cleopatra . . ."

"But, what good are flashbacks like this?" Karen asked. "Can they do any harm?"

"Not the kind you and I have had, Karen. If we have lived before, it is natural that, occasionally, vivid impressions stored in the deep-memory level are recalled. However, there is danger for the person who gets a fixation on the past that is false. Some people become so entranced with what they might have been in a former life that they neglect to become anything in this life. For example, I personally know of three women who claim they were Joan of Arc on a previous trip around. I am sure the count would grow to hundreds if we canvassed the country!"

Karen laughed. "I know," she agreed, "there are a lot of Joans and Cleopatras walking around—real wishful thinkers. But, if reincarnation is true, why *can't* I remember who I was?"

Karen's question is a disquieting one: "If I've lived before, why can't I remember previous lives?"

I reached for the dictionary on my desk and turned to the definition of *reincarnation,* which I read to Karen: *"The belief that the souls of the dead successively return to earth in new form or bodies, esp., a human body; hence, the belief in previous lives for the soul."*

I explained to Karen that the traditional concept of "previous lives" is really a misnomer. *You do not have previous lives, you have one life in continuous expression.* What you are today is a synthesis of all that you have ever been. You are today a composite of all the qualities, traits, concepts, cognitions, and values that you have accrued throughout your eons of being.

The person you are at the present has evolved from what you were in the past. Past qualities are not lost. They are assimilated into what you are today. Past glories and attainments are synthesized into powers latent in you today. Because of this assimilation process, specific and detailed memories of your life in the past are not necessary.

This does not mean, of course, that specific memories cannot be recalled. They can be and have been! No doubt, more such memories manifest in the dream state than we realize. Doubtlessly, valid memories of previous living have been recalled through regression during hypnosis.

But, there are many factors involved in such memory-recall that need to be examined.

In the first place, how clearly do you remember what you experienced just yesterday? Did the day's events register vividly enough with you to make a lasting impression? Or, were most of your hours filled with trivia and dull routine that left little on the memory scroll? Such data is not recallable.

In the second place, how accurately do you remember what you experienced yesterday? Too many people see experience through distorted eyes and store away memories that are inaccurate, negative, false, and self-defeating. Such data should *not* be recalled.

In the third place, think how cluttered your mind would become if you could consciously remember every hurt, every joy, every unhappiness, and every triviality that has befallen you since birth, much less in former incarnations! It is mercy that time distills your memory into an essence that becomes your present awareness. This essence is the consciousness you function with now, and be glad it is not cluttered with an eternity of extraneous memories!

To LIVE right now, live RIGHT now!

More important than remembering past incarnations is building present memories that will add constructive, creative, positive elements to the synthesis you must carry with you tomorrow, next week, and next life!

To reincarnate into a life beyond this time and place that is attractive, you must build qualities now that are to your credit. You are an evolving memory, and to remember rightly is to evolve.

What do I mean? If you fill your memory now with the hurts and slights of life, with unhappy experiences, and with hatreds engendered by misunderstanding and immaturity, you are blocking your mind's evolution. You force yourself to re-experience again and again the hurts and frustrations and humiliations with which your mind is filled.

On the other hand, if you fill your memory with what you have done in life that is worthy and inspiring, you will assimilate positive qualities into the distilled essence you are. Each new, positive addition to your memory-bank will raise you on the spiral of your own evolution. Failure will no longer recur, and you will find yourself climbing from one success to the next.

Now is the time of your life! Now is the time to build a positive memory. To *live* right now, you must live *right* now! Your unhappiness, if unhappiness you have, does not exist external to you. It is not due to the past, the way you have been treated, the environment into which you were born, the schooling you had, or the actions of congress. It is due to your memory of unhappiness.

The whole of your past, the present in which you live, and the potential days of your future are within you. A better future is dependent upon a better now. And, likewise, a better past is dependent upon a better now.

How to break the cyclicon of recurrence

Karen broke in, "What do you mean—a better past? How can my past be changed?"

"By your memory of it."

"How do I change my memory, then?" Karen persisted.

I explained to Karen the concept of the past, present, and future found in Chapter Four. Time is not a straight line connecting a yesterday that is over and a tomorrow that is not yet here. Rather, time is a track upon which your consciousness rolls. Within your consciousness you carry elements of the past into today and elements of today into the future.

Think of it this way: although each morning a new day dawns along the time-track, it will not seem new for you if you are rolling on in the old consciousness you brought with you from the past. If your thoughts are not new, old experiences recur for you with the cycle of each day.

Let us call this daily cycle of recurrence your CYCLICON. Picture yourself riding inside this cyclicon, reliving each day from the viewpoint of your well-worn state of mind. What will you see as you revolve round and round in your old, familiar consciousness? Old, familiar experiences!

How do you break the cyclicon pattern? How do you stop the carousel of recurrence? You change your consciousness! You change your memory of the past and your reactions to the present. Like attracts like, and you must think new thoughts to get new results.

Start with your memory of the past. After all, it may be more fancy than fact anyway. For example, within a single day, many events highlight the twenty-four hours. Perhaps a dozen separate things happen. You are the one who gives to these separate occurrences their value. Your reaction to one event may cause it to stand out, dwarfing all else by comparison.

Suppose that the thing which happened is of an undesirable nature—you are slighted or hurt; someone criticized you. This sticks in your memory. Even though other events are more positive, you remember this negative one. This distorted memory is now perpetuated in your consciousness. Hence, you live it not once, but many times as it revolves in your cyclicon of consciousness.

Here is the technique I gave Karen to eliminate repetitious memories of a negative nature. You can use it to re-evaluate reactions of today as well as memories of the past. Its purpose is to change the conditions of life by changing the mental state that chains you to a repetitious cycle of experience.

First: make it a practice to stop at the close of each day and re-evaluate the experiences you remember. Examine your responses to the events of the day. Did you react poorly to a thoughtless remark? Did your temper flare over some slight? Were you irritated as a motorist made a wrong turn in front of you? Were you sarcastic in something that you said? Did you act in an immature way?

As you go back over the events of the day—beginning with the last and going backward—use your imagination to relive them as they should have been lived. React in mind as you should have reacted in the flesh. What reaction would have made each experience more pleasant? How could you hvea handled yourself better? How could failure have been turned into success? In mind, visualize yourself responding in a more mature, masterful, successful manner.

This exercise in visualization will change the content of your cyclicon, and the next time that a similar event occurs, you will react from your corrected image.

Second: apply this technique to the more remote past. As it works for a single day, it will work for a longer span of time. Project yourself back in imagination five or ten years—or to any time that holds annoying memories for you. Visualize that past day as if it were the present.

Then, using visualization, relive those years as they should have been lived. Do not dwell on any vain regrets or guilt or resentment. Take what amounts to an impersonal look. View your actions and reactions from an expanded level of consciousness. Make your reactions *now* one of bigness and forgiveness, as a parent forgives a child. You are today the parent of the child you were yesterday—a much wiser parent. Forgive yourself for being that child!

"Do you mean to say," interrupted Karen, "that I can change the ways things happened?"

"I am not saying that you can change events that really took place, but you can change your response-pattern to these experiences—you can change their significance in your memory. You can prevent the cyclicon of recurrence from depositing you in like conditions today be altering what you permit to remain in your consciousness. Only a spiral can lead you out of a recurring cycle, and this depends upon the inner work you do on yourself."

Third: Use the following Psi-Programming Pointer to replace the image of *inept* reaction-patterns in the subconscious with constructive ones. With practice, you can change the cyclicon of recurrence into a spiral of new experience.

Ψ   Psi-Programming Pointer
THIS EVENING I RISE ON THE SPIRAL OF EXPANDED CONSCIOUSNESS AND REVIEW MY DAY'S PERFORMANCE, MENTALLY CORRECTING THOSE REACTIONS I COULD HAVE HANDLED IN A MANNER MORE MASTERFUL, SUCCESSFUL, AND MATURE.

The case of Mildred and her merry-go-round

There are many who are slaves to the cyclicon of recurrence and know it not! They go round and round each day on a carousel that deposits them at evening's end in the same place they started in the morning. Mildred O. was such a person.

Mildred was unhappy. Just to be in her presence was a most unrewarding experience. She seemed to carry about with her a sense of impending doom.

If Mildred had worn a placard around her neck announcing her misery, it would not have been more obvious than her downcast look, the droop of her jaw, and the dejected movement of her body. She was a walking advertisement of failure.

As Mildred sat across the desk from me, having been urged to come by a friend, I thought to myself, "Here is a woman who has just gone fifteen rounds with life and has lost every one." To my chagrin, I found myself voicing this remark. My visitor managed a wry smile and admitted that this was a good description.

"I have been on a merry-go-round all my life," she explained, "and I am getting tired of having the same failures repeat and repeat."

When a person begins to recognize recurring patterns of experience, there is hope, for change is then possible. So, I encouraged Mildred to tell me something about herself.

"My family was poor," Mildred related. " I was the first of seven children. My mother was an embittered woman and my father a drunkard. I guess you could say I was a chip from two gnarled blocks. Being the first child, most of the work fell to me, so I was not able to attend school beyond the fifth grade."

Mildred married young to get away from home. But, the man she married was very much like her father, and she soon divorced him. She married again, with the same end-result. For a third time, she tried marriage, and divorce occurred again. Now, she was contemplating a fourth husband. The recurrence of so many marital failures, however, made her hesitate.

In between husbands, Mildred worked in the restaurant field. Here, too, she demonstrated a recurrence pattern, beginning and ending one job after another in her predictable failure-style. She was caught in the cyclicon of recurrence! She had started no place, had been no place, and was going no place!

I explained to Mildred that her experiences had carved deep memory traces upon the subconscious mind "Regrettably, those memories that you call past experiences are not past. They move along with you in time. They stay in your consciousness. It is almost as if you made an appointment with memory to let your life revolve within the same general experience again. As long as the image of marital failure stays in your memory, you are asking for another divorce."

"But," Mildred declared, "won't the time come when I'll be happy?"

"You could live to be as old as Methuselah and *time* will not bring happiness. It is the *pattern in your consciousness* that makes your day a happy or unhappy experience. It is the memory of failure that causes failure to recur. For example, in psychosomatic medicine today, it is understood that memory of illness may help re-create the illness experienced. Likewise, the memory of unhappiness forms a track upon which unhappiness continues to run its appointed rounds."

Preventing the past from corrupting the present

To help Mildred understand how memory of the past reaches into today to make experience what it is, I compared the flow of consciousness along the memory-track to a river.

One of my earliest recollections is of a river, for my family lived on the Wabash. I can remember gathering shells along the bank and just sitting to look at the flow of the stream.

Like me, you have probably sat by a river and watched it. Your feeling may have been that as the water runs by it disappears, or does it? It flows out to sea, yes. But, then, it is lifted up becoming clouds, drifts back over the land, falls as rain or snow, and joins the flowing stream again.

Your consciousness is much like the water in the stream. It flows between the banks of your experience. Along the river bank are houses, trees, fields, and mountains. Along the banks of the stream-of-time are the experiences that constitute the scenery of your life—experiences of happiness and unhappiness; success and failure; love and loneliness. Which ones do you remember and carry along with you down to the sea?

Like the water that is lifted up above the land—to fall again and run its course back to the sea—at the end of the day you are lifted above time. Distilled as a part of your consciousness is your memory of the banks through which your waters-of-experience have run. Your consciousness next day runs its course again. Once again, familiar scenery is repeated.

If you have learned to be unhappy, your memory will carve the channel of unhappiness deeper and deeper with every run. If you have failed before, failure will recur with each cycling journey back to the sea.

However, if you have learned to be positive, optimistic, considerate, understanding, and appreciative of the opportunities that are yours, the scenery-of-your-life will be a joy to behold.

Each morning as you rejoin the time-track, you descend into time-space conditions like unto the ones previously experienced. This does not mean, however, that you must continue to ride the same carousel of recurrence. It is your prerogative to change the thoughts you have entertained and to reprogram your mind with new concepts. *This is the whole purpose of the day.*

Don't live for the time when things will change for you. Instead, change things for yourself by using the time you have today. Live right now, by living *right* now! Use each tick of the clock to make a new beginning for yourself. It is not the experience of sleep or death that changes a person, it is the experience of life!

Mildred promised me that she would do some positive work on herself each day. She was to begin by breaking the attitude of unhappiness that had become habitual, replacing her frowns and sighs with an occasional smile. She was to correct her negative thought-pattern. She was to replace words of complaint with words of optimism. She was to end each day a little happier, a little more confident and self-assured than she began.

"Mildred," I said, "it is not easy to break a merry-go-round of experience. You'll find you don't jump off it. You can, however, turn your carousel into a spiral, ending each cycling day somewhat higher and more positive than you started. Gradually, you'll climb up in consciousness to a new world of experience!"

I gave Mildred a Psi-Programmer similar to the one that follows. She used it to direct her subconscious mind each morning and throughout the day whenever her memory of past failure began to nag her. You, too, will find it effective in freeing yourself from an undesirable recurrence pattern.

Ψ   Psi-Programming Pointer

EACH TICK OF THE CLOCK IS A NEW BEGINNING FOR ME! NOTHING FROM MY PAST CAN TAKE PRECEDENCE OVER MY PRESENT. I PROGRAM MY MIND NOW WITH NEW THOUGHTS OF SUCCESS AND A NEW CYCLE OF EXPERIENCE BEGINS!

The art of living right now!

It was some time before I heard from Mildred again. When she did return to my office, I hardly knew her. The air of dejection was gone; her features were pleasant; even her posture had improved.

"Can you guess why I'm here?" Mildred asked.

"No, why?"

"We want you to be the one to marry us. Yes," Mildred nodded, "I'm getting married for the fourth time, but I've traded my merry-go-round for a spiral. This time it will be different!"

I believed her! There was a new maturity and self-assurance about her now, and I felt certain that she had broken free of the old memory of marital failure (the old cyclicon of recurrence).

"I know I can make this marriage a happy experience," Mildred concluded, "for I have learned the art of being happy *right* now!"

The larger cycle of birth and death

It is true, of course, that if you live *right* now, you are doing your best to provide for the present and the future. The memory pattern you build now is the distilled essence which you bring back with you to each day—to each life.

The larger cycle of birth and death is not unlike the daily cycle of morning and night. At death, you are lifted temporarily above time. You do not cease to be.

You are one life in continuous expression and re-expression. The consciousness, qualities, and attributes you accumulate are assimilated at death and re-express as your uniqueness when the time comes to run the course again. This is reincarnation; this is cyclic continuity as advanced by the Science of Higher Sense Perception.

The grand architect of birth is also the designer of what is spoken of as death. Therefore, if the one is good, the other must also be good. Life, in its total meaning, includes death—that phase when man is lifted above time as he knows it.

How to escape fear of death

"You speak so convincingly of the continuity of life, but how can you be so sure it continues?" the woman in her late forties was saying.

I knew Bertha G. was deeply troubled about something, and I encouraged her to talk.

"Well," she explained, "I've never thought too much about death, but Tuesday I am going to the hospital for an operation and, frankly, I am scared."

I asked her about the operation and learned that it was a rather common one which she should not fear.

"I suppose," she explained, "that my concern is due to an experience I had about ten years ago. I had another operation then which was considered minor, and I almost died. Now, facing this one, I find myself worrying about the end. What happens at death? Where do you go? What's the purpose of it all?"

"Bertha," I replied, "one time the great mystic, Jacob Boehme, was asked where the soul went at death. He answered by saying that there was no need for it to go anywhere."

As Bertha listened, I explained that the real Self is an entity that exists beyond time and space. The four dimensions of length, breadth, height, and time belong to the physical body, not to the real You. The real Self lives in eternity now, and if you were fully conscious of that Self, you would be functioning on the fifth dimension. On the fifth dimension, past, present, and future may be embraced in one glance. Hence, there is no need for the real Self to go anywhere. It is already there. The need is to become *conscious* of that Self you really are.

"Is that the purpose of death," Bertha inquired.

"No, it's the purpose of life!"

"Doesn't death interrupt that purpose, then?" she asked.

"It is true that growth in consciousness takes place through living," I replied, "but the phase called death facilitates *the assimilation of growth.*"

I then traced for Bertha the process of assimilation found in nature. You can see it at work in the evolution of species into higher forms. You can see it in the annual cycle of growth and dormancy in deciduous trees. You can see it in the rhythmic response of flowering bulbs to the seasons of spring and fall. Everywhere you look, you can see a process of outbreathing and inbreathing taking place—a process of expression and assimilation.

Think of *outbreathing* as life expressing (pressing out) into form. Think of *inbreathing* as life leaving a particular form.

For you, that outbreathing of life is the real Self expressing through the vehicle of your physical body in order to develop your *conscious* mental powers. To develop consciously, you must come in contact with the objective time-space world.

Imagine that each incarnation is a laboratory into which the *chemist* of the real Self goes for the purpose of conducting experiments in the refinement of conscious awareness. The laboratory of experience for one person may be rural farm life. For another, it may be the challenge of crowded city life. For still another, it may be the crucible of a primitive caste system.

Next comes the inbreathing process. Now the *chemist* leaves the lab to assimilate the experiments that have been conducted. Figuratively speaking, he goes over the formulas, work sheets, and tests involved. He digests and incorporates the lessons learned. "Ah! Here is something of value; it will become a part of the distilled wisdom retained. Ah! Here is a lesson not quite completed. More work remains to be done on it next time. I can hardly wait to get back to my lab!"

Then the outbreathing process takes place again to enable the eternal Self to carry on more experiments in *conscious awakening* and *conscious self-discovery*. In short, the chemist survives the laboratory and moves on to a new lab to continue the work of refinement of conscious powers.

You *can* take it with you!

Through the assimilation process, the qualities and attributes you have accumulated become a permanent part of you. You *can* take it with you!

The story is told of two men watching a funeral procession for a wealthy man of the community. At the end of the procession, a number of vans, trucks, and assorted vehicles were following slowly, waiting for the cortege to turn off to the cemetery.

It so happened that the first vehicle tied up in traffic behind the procession was an armored truck. The two men watching the cortege eyed the truck with surprise, and one remarked to the other, "So, he is really taking it with him after all!"

What is it that a person takes with him? Most certainly, he does not take stocks and bonds. He does not take acres of land or physical beauty. He does not take money or jewelry. Although, there *is* a provoking thought in a report of the man who, after reading *The Search for Bridey Murphy*, changed his will and left everything to himself.

What will you take with you into the tomorrows of life? Can you take with you anything other than that which you are?

If you have a consciousness of supply, this you will take with you, for *this* you are. Of course, you cannot take stocks and bonds; you cannot take physical wealth. But what is physical wealth other than the effect of consciousness? And, a wealth-producing consciousness must continue to manifest like effects.

If you have a consciousness of love, your love will produce effects that belong to it. If you have a consciousness of beauty, of appreciation, of compassion, etc., the same is true. No matter what your state of mind, you will take it with you and it will produce at its own level, for *this* you are!

"That seems logical," Bertha concluded. "And I suppose the same is true of a negative consciousness."

"It is," I said. "But this is something you don't need to worry about, Bertha. Aside from the fear you told me of today, I've always seen the kind of positive qualities in you that will produce happiness wherever you are."

I answered Bertha's final question by explaining that one of the first functions of consciousness is to produce effects that belong to it. Broadly, each one attracts what belongs to him. That *belonging* may be not only in terms of what he deserves but also in terms of what he needs.

However, so long as the consciousness stays the same, it cannot produce different results. It goes round and round in the same recurrence cycle. It follows the same river banks down to the sea each time.

If a person keeps company with a failure-pattern, his consciousness cannot produce success as a result. He will continue to build a life patterned after his dominant state of mind until he changes it.

For example, driving through the coal-mining district of West Virginia years ago, you could find many small towns built by

[1]Bernstein, Morey, *The Search for Bridey Murphy*. New York: Doubleday & Company, Inc., 1956.

mining companies. Every house looked alike because the same blueprint was used in its construction. Similarly, it may be said that a person's consciousness is a company of thoughts, ideas, beliefs, and attitudes. They register as a rate of vibration which externalizes outwardly in experiences that are remarkably alike. Unless a person changes his mental blueprint, how can the results be different?

How to activate the law of recurrence

To stay as you are with the same likes and dislikes, the same attitudes, the same prejudices and fears, is to recur without change.

Why is this so? Well, just as a *company* house takes the form that the blueprint gives it (and every house built from the same blueprint will look alike), so will your blueprint of awareness outpicture as a *company* life until you change the plans.

Now, recurrence is easy to come by. If you want your life to recur as it has been, if you want to keep riding the cyclicon of repetition down the time-track, here are a number of things to do·

1. Don't listen to new ideas.
2. Don't develop new interests.
3. Don't let anyone interfere with yo ir right to gripe, to worry, and to complain.
4. Keep your present attitudes and prejudices intact.
5. Remember how terribly people have always treated you.
6. Blame others for your state of affairs.
7. Keep your memory of hurts and humiliations vivid.
8. Insist that you are always right, and bristle with indignation when others criticize you.
9. Give advice freely, and insist that others conform to your standards.
10. Persist in an illusion that tomorrow will be better without doing anything today to improve it.

Do these things and you will spin like a top in the same place. And how long will the top spin? Until there is a change in the tone of your consciousness.

Using the key to life today

The key to life is in your hand today. Its use is up to you. If you hold it idly and use it not, the Science of Higher Sense Perception can do you little good. To demonstrate the success and fulfillment this Science affords, you must put the key in the door, unlock it, and begin your ascent in consciousness.

The rungs of the stairway to HSP power lie before you, but no one can demonstrate from any rung other than that on which he stands. You cannot tap the powers that belong to the fifth dimension while standing on the fourth rung. You can, however, step up to the fifth by realizing that the higher rung exists and by using the techniques, formulas, and methods presented in this book.

Now that you have read the *Science of Higher Sense Perception*, go back over the Psi-Programming Pointers and HSP Sensitivity Training Techniques described and use them daily in your life.

No one can grow for you, nor can anyone *make* you grow. But you can, through study, application, and action, step up to higher rungs on the spiraling stairway to personal achievement.

Now, train yourself to accept the good that can be yours at each level of experience—the physical, mental, emotional, and expanded-aware ess level—by following this final HSP Sensitivity Tehcnique:

HSP SENSITIVITY TRAINING TECHNIQUE NO. 10

LIVING FULLY THIS DA'

You seat yourself comfortably in the chair yo.' have used in sessions past. You relax and let go of all tension. (After reading this three times, close your eyes and mentally affirm the following:)

You are a beneficiary of life. You are heir to what it is. As that beneficiary, you share in all the riches latent to the four levels of experience—the physical, mental, emotional, and expanded-awareness level.

In your mind's eye, see yourself at the first level. It is represented by the main floor of a magnificent mansion. A glistening white marble staircase rises before you and around you are tables laden with treasure chests. These riches are but tokens. In your awareness, you know they symbolize the bounty of nature, the wealth in the bowels of the earth, and the natural resources the universe spreads before you.

You rejoice in the abundance that surrounds you on the physical level. True, it is a level of "things," but it is not to be despised. You accept your heritage, and a feeling of deep gratitude wells up within you as you silently affirm, *"The wealth of this day is mine!"*

You turn your gaze now to the spiraling marble staircase before you. It leads to higher levels of yourself. In your imagination, you climb to the second floor of the mansion—the mental level. You look about you and find that you are in a library whose shelves are lined with books, blueprints, patterns, musical scores, sketches, and drawings. You feel ideas flooding your mind, impinging upon your consciousness, and inspiring you to startling achievements.

You realize that you are in the room of the intellect. You are heir to this vast library of ideas and to the ability to reason, perceive, analyze, deduce, synthesize, and utilize its wisdom. You claim your mental heritage and joyously accept the guidance it holds for you, saying silently, *"The wisdom of this day is mine!"*

You turn your footsteps back again to the staircase. In your mind's eye, you climb to the third floor of the mansion—the emotional level. The decor of the hall you enter now is warm and harmonious. It is something you feel more than see. It is a radiance enclosing you. It is the warm embrace of universal love. You recognize that you are in the hall of feeling—the empathy, warmth, affection, appreciation, accord, and love that give value to life.

You know a deep peace, a harmony that unites you in understanding with mankind, and a kinship with life that is overpowering. You accept your heritage of the heart, silently saying, *"The love of this day is mine!"*

You face the staircase again and continue your ascent. You find yourself now on the fourth floor of the mansion—the expanded-awareness level. A feeling of awe surges over you as you behold this realm. Here you experience precognition and retro-cognition for you are above time. Here you are clairvoyant for you can see all things clearly. Here all causation originates. It is the realm of First Cause! You realize that the other levels are subservient to this, the higher dimension.

You are heir to this realm for that which you are had its origin here. You claim the expanded powers of this level and the dominion it gives you over the physical, mental, and emotional affairs of life, silently declaring, *"Expanded-awareness is now mine!"*

Your vision next enlarges and you see the mansion as a whole. The four floors are an integral, balanced part of the entire structure. You are the dweller of the mansion. It is your House-of-Self. In it, you feel fulfilled, secure, and at peace. Over the hearth of your heart, these words appear: "MY CUP RUN-NETH OVER." They become your talisman, your motto forever-more. And, you declare:

And so it is!

SUMMARY CAPSULES

YOUR MEMORY OF YESTERLIVES

Resident within you and inscribed upon the memory scroll of mind are experiences of yesterday, yesteryear, and yesterlives. However, specific memories of the past would only burden you with cluttered details and are not essential. They are assimilated into what you are today—a synthesis of all the qualities, traits, and values you have accrued through the eons of being. The person you *were* is the person you *are*, with today added.

YOU, A CONTINUOUS EXPRESSION

You do not have many lives, but one life in continuous expression. This is reincarnation! Just as now each morning you awaken with the assimilated wisdom of the day before, so in the larger cycle of life you awaken to the dawning of a new expression with the distilled essence of all you have accumulated to date. You are today the reincarnated off-spring of all your yesterdays and the parent of all your tomorrows.

THE TIME OF YOUR LIFE

Today is the *time* in which you live. This is your moment of change—this is your moment of destiny. You are changed not through dying but through living! This is the moment to re-evaluate your memory record. This is the time to alter your consciousness and improve your self-image. Postpone it no longer! There is no other time for you than *now*—always it will be NOW. This is the time of your life—LIVE!

YOU CAN TAKE IT WITH YOU

Not only can you take it with you, you must take it with you! You cannot escape what you are, but you can always become more. Become more alert, more discerning, more considerate, more masterful, and this *more* will register on the scroll of mind and accrue to you as legal tender wherever you are in this universe. It will purchase for you values equal to your currency-of-consciousness anywhere.

BREAK YOUR CYCLICON OF RECURRENCE

Until consciousness changes, experience remains the same. Patterns of thought recur along the time-track until the course is altered. To break the cyclicon of recurrence, you must change the awareness in which you revolve day after day. You must step out into new mental territory. You must step up to new plans, new thought patterns, new aspirations. You must trade your merry-go-round for an upward spiral!